Weigh and See: How I Lost 35 Pounds in 4 Months

CARLO RICCI, PhD

DEDICATION

As always, first, to Gina, Annabel, and Karina who I love unconditionally. And, to all those who are looking to lose weight and get healthier, may this inspire you and make your life better.

CONTENTS

ACKNOWLEDGMENTS

In writing this book I have benefited tremendously from people who were kind enough to review my book and offer me formal feedback. Among these people, I would like to thank Gina Luongo, OCT, MEd; John Vitale, PhD; Christine Cho, PhD; Ellie Berger, PhD; Steven Taylor, OCT, MEd; Melissa Bock, a Nurse Practitioner; and Tammy Dwyer, Nurse. I have also benefited from many informal conversations with people and would like to thank them for their insights and the inspiration that the conversations stimulated in me. I value their insights.

1 WHY I DECIDED TO DIET

The secret to losing weight with the goal of getting healthier is not much of a secret; simply put, eat less and make healthier choices. We all know this to be the case, yet so many of us find it so hard to follow this simple proven road to successful weight loss and improved health. In part, this book hopes to build confidence, motivate, and inspire those interested to lose weight and get healthier by sharing what I did to lose weight with the help of an inexpensive scale that I bought on sale for $9.99 at my local retailer. What I am hoping to get across is that my message is more than simply about weight loss. It is about getting healthy, and one way of doing that is to eat smarter, which I define as eating nutritious food, and the right portion size. I think too many of us overeat and do so without understanding what a portion size is, and how much food we actually need in a day.

For years I knew that fluctuating within 7 pounds of the

1

weight I was, meant that I was about 35 pounds overweight, mostly around my mid-section. Despite knowing this, I did little about it. In truth, I was not too bothered about it and as long as I maintained that weight I was fine with it.

The first and most important step in transitioning to a healthier me was deciding that I was no longer fine with the status quo. After having some conversations with medical professionals and others, I decided that it was time to change. Medically, I am fine, but was not sure at the time, and that uncertainty was all the impetus I needed to decide to make a change.

So, after consulting with professionals and doing some research, I decided what is a healthy weight for me. I decided that I would get to my goal weight, remain at that weight for awhile to see how healthy I felt at that weight, and then reassess if necessary. The rest of this book is the story of how I accomplished that in just over four months.

Although in the title I allude to the concept of diet and throughout the book I use the words weight loss, I need to say at the outset that these words in isolation are not the best words for what I am trying to get at in this book. I use those words because ultimately they are the words we use to describe weight loss. In part, this book is clearly about how to diet and lose weight, but it is also about so much more. More importantly, it is about becoming a healthier person and adopting a lifestyle change. To me the term diet implies a short term plan we embark on to get to a certain goal. I have seen far too many people on diets fail, and what I am trying to impart is a lifestyle change that leads to better health. So when I use the word diet and weight loss, please keep in mind that I am using them to mean a permanent lifestyle change that results in better health.

Among the terms I use to call this approach to healthy dieting is data driven dieting, or evidence based dieting, or willed dieting, or self-determined dieting, or weigh and see dieting to better health. The word "diet" is a short form for the health professional use of the phrased intention of weight loss diet.

To clarify, when I use the terms evidence based and data driven dieting, what I mean is that each of us needs to make our commitment to better health personal. So I use the terms evidence based and data driven to mean that I stand on the scale daily and use that data as evidence to drive my goal of achieving better health. In addition, I also consult with professionals (medical doctors, for example) and use the data and evidence they gather through blood work and other measures to make sure that I feel comfortable doing what I am doing and that it is indeed leading to better health.

My PhD is in education and learning, and so I am

approaching dieting using this lens. I am also a researcher who relies on evidence and data and so these are also central to this approach to healthy weight loss.

The ultimate goal is not to lose weight, or to keep losing more and more weight; nor is the idea, the more weight I lose the better. But the goal is to get to a healthy weight given my body type, age, height, and other measures that might be relevant to each individual case. This is why for many it would be advisable to do personal research, and in consultation with professionals, to determine what is a healthy weight.

As an academic, I appreciate the importance of research. Of course there are many types of research methodologies and for this book I have decided to use narrative or autobiographical research as my guide. Furthermore, as a staunch believer in the willed curriculum and willed learning, I know people can teach themselves to follow their own way to better health. In the book I also try hard to show my appreciation for the work that professionals in the field contribute to helping us understand how to become healthier. They help us define what it means to be a healthy individual, as well as a healthy community. Of course, this is at times contentious and so each of us has to work to define what healthy means to us, given our unique body, mind, spirit, and emotions.

As an aside, my grocery bill is also much less now than it was before I started to eat smarter. The reason I share this is because it is an indication that I am consuming less food, and the upside is the less food we consume collectively, the more there would potentially be to share with others. So, if more and more people get healthier, and collectively we consume, waste, and throw out less food, there could hopefully be a social benefit.

What I Used To Do

Before I started on this path to better health, what I did to maintain my weight was to stand on a scale every Friday and to make sure that my weight stayed the same from week to week. In other words, I was maintaining my weight at a level that was higher than I knew it should be, but not so high that it concerned me—I cared enough to monitor but not enough to make a change. What I would do is eat less during the week and binge on the weekends, and by eating less during the week my weight would come down by the weekend and so my weight remained stable in the long term.

So, if I wanted to have a treat I would buy it and save it for the weekend. Knowing that I could eat whatever I wanted come the weekend, helped me remain disciplined during the week and this approach assisted me with keeping my weight stable. Once the weekend arrived, I would eat and eat. I would binge on boxes of ice-cream, chocolate, fast-food; essentially anything I desired.

It's important to note that even though I was eating less during the week, my food intake during the week was still more than what I needed. Nevertheless, by Friday I was back down to my then goal-weight and so I was happy with that, and really felt that it was working for me, and at the time, it was.

As age crept up on me, it became clear that my weekend binges coupled with eating less during the week were helping me maintain a certain weight, but that it was not doing my body any good was becoming clearer and clearer. Remember that during the week I was eating less than I did on the weekends, but still more than I actually needed. That is why, in part, overall I still remained overweight. As happens to many of us, age precipitates health concerns. After meeting with a few doctors, it became clear that I now needed to rethink my approach and my diet. Overall, I am and was even before I started my diet a fairly healthy person. I was and continue to do many of what medical experts consider the right things: I exercise, I do not smoke, I do not drink alcohol, I drink plenty of water, and I am a vegetarian. But admittedly, I was slightly overweight, which is something that I am glad that I have since corrected.

Now I want to be clear, I am not suggesting that everyone who weighs more than society suggests they should needs to lose weight. In fact, if you are happy with yourself, and if you feel good, and if there is no reason, medically or otherwise, for you to lose weight, then continue doing what you are doing. Also, I am not suggesting that losing weight will cure everyone's ills, but for many in the world we live in, weight loss is clearly the whole or part of the answer to better health.

Why I Am Writing This Book

As an academic and researcher and a believer in social justice, I am always looking for ways to help make the world a better place, and to find ways to help people in the world. In part, this book is another one of my humble attempts at doing that. After recently watching a documentary about cancer, I realized that being proactive, rather than reactive, makes a tremendous difference. So rather than only spending resources to find cures for people with cancer, cancer researchers and advocates decided to find ways to prevent people from getting cancer in the first place. Some cancers are genetic, but many are environmental.

So, the cancer researchers and advocates decided that they were raising tremendous amounts of money and that they were making some breakthroughs in finding cures and trying to beat cancer, but that one thing they were overlooking is advocating for people to stop behaving in ways that put them at high risk of getting cancer. Thankfully, once the message starting getting through that cigarettes, for example, cause cancer many, many lives were saved by convincing people to stop smoking in the first place. Similarly, I am hoping that this book can have analogous results.

So, for example, when the doctors, researchers, and activists recognized the connection between smoking cigarettes and cancer, they campaigned and made the public aware of this high risk behavior, and as more people listened and fewer people smoked, certain lung cancers, for example, noticeably decreased and lives were saved.

I want to be clear that I am not suggesting that if only we lived healthier lives, that that alone will ensure that we will not get sick. Furthermore, I am not suggesting that if we do get sick, it is our fault and we alone are to blame. Of course, I believe that this argument is blatantly false and unfair. As I see it, illnesses are a result of both genetics and the environment, and sometimes the best environment cannot trump genetics, but sometimes and in some cases it can. In addition, I do believe that regardless of our circumstances we can all benefit from living healthier lives. Ultimately, each of us needs to make our own decisions regardless of what I believe.

And so in my case, I cannot change my genetics or nature, but I can improve how I nurture myself, and I am not alone. Many of us are making ourselves ill by living a lifestyle that is harmful to our wellbeing. But by living a less harmful life, we can live healthier, and for those of us in that position, diet is a big part of the solution to better health. In part, I also wanted to lose weight in the hopes that I will be less of a burden on the health care system.

Better Health Through Dieting

In one of my other books titled *The Willed Curriculum, Unschooling, and Self-Direction: What Do Love, Respect, Trust, Care, and Compassion Have to do with Learning?* I write about the importance of love, trust, respect, care, and compassion and what it means in relation to learning. In this book I believe that this framework is central to weight loss. Love, I believe, figures centrally, and I am writing this book out of love. Love for my family members, for all of humanity, and the universe at large.

Far too many people I know are suffering from diabetes, high cholesterol, high blood pressure, have trouble walking, other mobility issues, and other illnesses. Again, not everyone who has these issues can reverse the effects through diet, but some can, and I truly believe that many of the people I am thinking of can reverse or at least better their health issues by improving their diet.

Food Made To Be Addictive

I know far too many people who have tried to lose weight and simply have failed. Some lose weight for awhile but the weight eventually comes back. Part of the problem is that many rely on gimmicks and fads, and gimmicks and fads are exactly that, gimmicks and fads. Ultimately, the only way to lose weight is to eat less and make healthier choices, and the only one who can do this is the individual. So I decided that I wanted to lose weight, and thereby I was motivated internally to do so. I decided that I would rather lose weight and get healthier than overindulge, and that decision factored enormously and made losing weight to get healthier a priority for me; without this decision it likely would not have happened. Food is made to taste so good that we can easily become prey to its deliciousness.

Consumption and Portion Size

In the capitalistic world we live in, the focus is on consumption and money: The more we consume and spend the better. This, of course, is self-evident in every aspect of the world we live in and mirrored in the food industry. Recently my wife and I were sitting in a shopping mall fast-food court waiting for our children and their friends. Given my new lens and awareness, I was struck by how unhealthy a lot of the food was that people were consuming, and how much they were given as portions. Even the healthier food option overfilled the trays with huge portions.

Portion sizes are grossly over inflated. How much we need to eat to sustain ourselves and to live a healthy life is way out of sync with practice, habit, custom, and tradition. When we watch television and movies we see huge portions; when we go to restaurants we see huge portions; and even in our homes we often get huge portions, and this all combines to falsely normalize what a meal is. By constantly getting bombarded and exposed to huge portion sizes, we begin to internalize that this is indeed what a portion size is. Of course, this cannot be further from the truth.

Broken Signals From The Body

What we actually need to eat and sustain ourselves is nowhere near the mounds and mounds of food that we see people consuming all around us. We have trained ourselves to overeat, and we need to train ourselves to eat what we need, not what we want. For many of us, the mechanism in our bodies that tells us how much food we need is broken, and so we need to temporarily stop listening to it until we fix it through retraining.

As a young person growing up I was always made to finish what was on my plate, even if my body was telling me I was full. I was trained by my family modeling and largely by popular culture to ignore what my body was saying and to listen to my parents and popular culture, who I see as the external authority. In this case it is clear to me now that they were wrong to force-feed me and that I was right to resist. I now have to retrain my body and retrain myself to listen to my body, and thereby regain this ability.

In the meantime, I have decided not listen to my body when it tries to tell me that I need more food than I actually need by signaling to me that I am still hungry. I have decided to ignore it, and to temporarily use my mind to override what my body is telling me, as long as I know that I am getting the correct amount of nutrients by consulting with dietitians and doctors, if I feel the need to.

So if I know that I have to have three meals a day, and if I know what a portion size is, and what healthy food is, then I can use that to determine what I should have for breakfast, lunch, dinner, and a few snacks in between.

I know I need to have three meals a day (and snacks) and for each meal I have to eat good food and make sure that it is an appropriate portion size. If I am doing this and my body is telling me I am hungry, then I need to question it, and to maybe walk away and see if after some time I am still hungry. Most of the times when I do this, it turns out that I was not hungry after all. Conversely, if I am not eating enough and my body is telling me that I do not need anymore food, then I have to reflect on this as well. I will do this until my body is "fixed" and it shows me that it can be trusted again to tell me when I am hungry and when I am full.

As I am retraining my body to correctly signal whether I am hungry or not, I am learning that the less I eat, the less I want to eat, and that as my body is readjusting I am becoming more capable of listening to it. In the process I am becoming more attuned to what my body needs, rather than being tempted by the deliciousness of food and the consumption mentality. When I am full, I am full, and being full does not mean feeling stuffed. Retraining myself to redefine what it means to be full is a big part of what I, and many of us, need to do. By redefine I mean that we need to be more mindful of how to become healthier, in this case by making smarter decisions, which for many of us means eating smaller portions and healthier more nutritious foods. In other words, feeling stuffed or overindulging is not what being full means. Being full means that we eat the right amount and type of food that we need to be healthy.

Learning To Say No

Learning to say no when I am full is a lesson I owe to my two wonderful children, and I am indebted to them for living their wisdom for me. As a parent, I believe in self-determination and so my children (born in 2003 and 2005) have more freedom than most other children I know. In short, they determine what they want to eat, when, how much and so on, and this has always been the case for them. They have always been allowed to listen to their bodies, and interestingly enough they stop eating when they are full, not when they are stuffed. In fact, they often pass on desserts and other food and simply say they are passing on the food because they are full and they do not feel like having it. In part, I believe that this is likely because they know they can have it whenever they want, and it is not a special treat for them so they are not "missing" out. There is always a next time and they decide when that next time is, and so having more freedom to make these decisions results in them feeling more empowered. If they did not have this freedom and they had to rely on my authority, then I imagine that it would be harder for them to say no to accepting a treat. It would be hard for them not to accept a treat because they do not know when I or an external authority will be so generous next, and so they better have it now because who knows when the next time an external authority will allow them to indulge.

Force-Feeding

Many children I know are made to eat all of their food before they can have dessert, and so they overeat on their food since they were forced to eat what someone else made them, rather than what they actually needed or wanted. In addition, then they add to that by overeating on dessert. Consequently, first, they are trained to have dessert even though they are full and, second, they are trained to have as much as they can because they might not be able to eat it at another time. They might very well think that this is it, it is available and so binge now because they might not get a chance later.

Saying No To Treats And Food

So, my children have taught me that you can say no to "treats" or all types of food if you are full. I recall times when I would take them to a store and ask them if they wanted to get a chocolate bar or some other treat, and they would say no thank you. I recall thinking to myself are you serious, are you children? How can you turn down a treat? What powerful lessons from such wise beings.

They have also taught me what a portion size is. They almost always leave food on their plate, and over the years we have all become better and better at making less and less since we know how much they eat. Very few times we underestimated how hungry they were and admittedly did not make enough food, and they simply supplemented with something else. We always have plenty of food in the house and they are always welcome to have whatever they desire. When they are full, they are full and that is that.

Portion Size

I am trying to understand how little food I actually need and am doing so with the help of an inexpensive $9.99 scale. Once I began to love weight loss and better health more than food, I knew that I was well on my way. I am approaching this not as a medical doctor, or a dietitian, or a weight control expert, but simply as an average person trying to get to a healthy weight. Having said that, I recognize that the concept of a healthy weight is very difficult to explain. There are so many things to consider (personal, societal, political, and so on). Ultimately, I believe it is up to the individual to decide, when they feel healthiest, and sometimes in consultation with a professional.

So my message is not technical but simple: to lose weight you need to eat less and better; and only you can do it, no one can lose the weight for you; and until you really, really want to do it, you never will. As I say throughout the book, eating less is a significant part of weight loss, but eating the right foods cannot be overlooked.

In what follows I will share with you more about what I did to lose the weight. I want to make it clear that what I did is not the only way. The specifics of what worked for me may not work for you. The foods I like, for example, may not be the foods you like. The strength and beauty of this approach to weight loss and better health is that there are infinite possibilities and one constant. The constant is that the scale does not lie. So like a researcher I need to modify what I do based on what the scale tells me. I know that it will not lie to me, and if I listen to it, better health will follow.

Of course, ultimately a $9.99 scale should not be considered the master, but being healthy should. After reading a draft of the book, a friend commented with the following, "For example, someone who is anorexic could still be trying to lose weight based on the fact that the scale tells them that they are too heavy. But, they are ignoring that loved ones and friends are telling them they are too skinny and unhealthy as a result." He goes on to ask, "Where do you place your trust? In a scale? Or, in what your family and friends are telling you?" Frankly, I believe that in cases where people are becoming less healthy your trust should be placed with your family and friends and other professionals. Remember, the goal is to become healthier and not simply to lose weight. In some cases losing weight can mean that you are becoming less healthy. So, as a friend aptly said, "for me the scale is a tool, not a master."

2 STANDING ON A SCALE

If what you are doing is working, then keep doing it. If you are happy with your current health then do nothing. It may catch up to you and it may not, so keep rolling the dice, and spinning the wheel and let's sincerely hope for the best. If, however, you need to lose weight I will share with you what I did, and I hope you find it helpful, and worthwhile, and that you will adopt it and make it your own.

Deciding To Lose Weight And Get Healthy

First, I had to make the decision that this is something that I wanted to do, and a discussion with my doctors was the kick-start that I needed. Once I decided that I would lose weight and get healthy rather than overeat, I was well on my way. Again, I am not a medical doctor or a dietitian or an expert in weight loss. I am simply an average person looking to lose weight. Throughout this book I will not be providing fancy formulas or jargon, but a simple, easy strategy that anyone can do and that works for me.

Seeking Expert Advice

Given that I am not a weight loss professional, I strongly recommend that before you embark on such an impactful, health-altering lifestyle that you take the time to consult a supportive professional and see what, if anything, they can advise. After all, the idea is to become more and not less healthy. Also, be sure to take your time and to see it as a marathon and not a short sprint. What I mean is that this will take time, and so my advice is do it right and do it gradually. Start by slowly decreasing your food intake and stand on the scale to see the results. If you do not see results then continue to decrease your food intake until you begin to get the results you want to achieve. Again, decreasing food intake is fine, but one still has to eat the right foods in order to retain nutritional balance.

Binging

Once I decided that I wanted to do this, the next thing I did was that I cut out my binge weekends. That for me was a huge part of it and admittedly it was something that I was not sure I could do. I was binging on the weekend for so many years that I thought that I was dependent on it. I truly believed that this was the magic wand that allowed me to stay so faithful the rest of the week. I believed that weekend binging allowed me to eat less during the week so that I could keep to my then weight goal. At some level I knew that I was still overweight, but it was a weight that I was happy with and had I not had a medical "worry" to change, I likely would have happily continued doing what I was doing.

At times, people would comment that I was carrying some extra fat around my midsection and depending on what clothes I would wear, the obviousness of it would change. So I knew that I was and it was confirmed occasionally by others.

My weekend binges were so overindulgent that for me eliminating the binges made a big difference towards better health and weight loss. During my weekend binge days, I would often eat more in one meal than I would the rest of the week.

Short-Term Goals, Long-Term Goals, And Milestones

The beauty of data driven weight loss as I define it, is in its simplicity. All I need to do is stand on the scale at the same time everyday and if the reading is higher than I want it to be, then I need to eat less in order to achieve my desired new short-term-goal. A short-term-goal is the realistic weekly number I aim to achieve as I work my way toward long-term-goal. For example, if I currently weigh 167 pounds and my long-term-goal is to be 140 pounds, then in-between I would set short-term-realistic goals as I work toward my long-term-goal. For instance, I step on the scale on a Friday and I weigh 167 pounds, my short-term-goal could be that by the following Friday I will be at 165 pounds. If I am lower than that, and I feel healthy, and I am eating healthy foods, then there is nothing to worry about and I know that what I am doing is working. If I am above that number, or the same weight come the following Friday, then I know that I have to simply eat less to achieve my goal.

As I said in the beginning and all along, my goal is to get healthier and so, for example, after I sit at 140 pounds for awhile and if I feel less healthy rather than healthier, then I should be prepared to reassess. In my case, I am not feeling immediate adverse health effects from the weight loss, but if over time adverse health effects materialize because of my weight loss, I will simply add more weight until I determine that I am at a healthy weight.

It is important to note that what I found most useful is a daily weigh-in so that I have frequent data to help me monitor what I am doing. In my case I weigh myself every morning and without any clothes on so that I can get the most accurate reading—you may not think so, but clothes can skew the results by a number of pounds. Hence the title, *Weigh and See.* I weigh myself and see the results.

Along with my long-term goal, I also find it helpful to have intermediate-goals or milestones. So to recap using the example I gave above, if I weigh 167 pounds, and my long-term goal is to reach 140 pounds, and in between I have set the short-term goal of losing about 2 pounds a week, so by the following week rather than weighing 167, my short-term goal is to weigh 165 pounds. In addition to my long-term goal of reaching 140 pounds and my short-term goal of 165 pounds, I also have milestones that I find helped keep me motivated, so milestones could be that I can't wait to break 160 pounds, and then 155 pounds, and then 150 pounds and so on. So milestones, I find are additional points that help keep me motivated on my way to my long-term goal. Again, I am simply sharing what worked for me and if this does not seem helpful for you, then simply modify and do what you feel works better.

I found that having a long-term-goal, and short-term-goals, and intermediate-goals or milestones was a great way to keep me motivated. Rather than one large goal that takes months and months to achieve, having these smaller realistic goals made me feel that I was accomplishing very positive results. The goals gave me something to strive for and really helped to keep me motivated. When I reached my goals and milestones, I really felt a sense of accomplishment and I was on a definite high.

Celebration

To recap then, a long-term-goal is the weight I actually want to be, and in the above example it was 140 pounds. A short-term-goal is how much I want to lose from week to week, and in the above example I started off at 167 pounds and at the end of the first week I wanted to be at less than 165 pounds. A milestone along the way from the current weight to the long-term-goal could be wanting the scale to read below 165, and then 160, and then 155, and so on. Each of the short-term goals and milestones are cause for celebration as I work to reach my long-term goal.

Again, simplicity for me is the key. Like a researcher I stand on the scale everyday and if the number is higher than it should be, then I know I have to eat less; if the number is recurrently the same, then I know I have to eat less; if the number is lower than the previous day, or days, or week, then I know that I am on track.

Learning About My Body

I have learned a lot about my body and how it reacts to the consumption of various food types, and amounts. By weighing myself everyday, I am able to see the impact that my previous days eating has on my overall weight and I am able to adjust accordingly. There is no greater feeling than setting a realistic goal and reaching it. Weighing myself everyday also allows me to correct and catch overeating quickly, and that allows me to modify and change what I am doing so that by the end of the week I am where I want to be.

I recognize that scale weight does not only indicate body fat, and that the scale is allowing me to see variances in things such as water retention and bowel movements. A person does not gain fat in a day. So, although I realize that body fat is not gained and lost in a day, the scale is my accountability that reminds me to keep eating what I need, and not as much as I want.

The idea is to lose the weight gradually and honestly. Again, the scale does not lie to me and I should not lie to others or to myself. What I caution is that gaming the system might work in the short term, but it will not help create the good habits I will likely need to sustain weight loss. So, for example, eating a lot for a few days and then "starving" myself for a couple so that I will reach my short-term goal at the end of the week does not sound like a healthy and sustainable plan. This might help me reach my short-term goal once, but if I continue to eat large portions and then try to "starve away" some weight I will not be able to lose enough to reach my milestones or long-term goals, since overall I am still overeating, and so I will gain and lose, gain and lose, only to a certain point, and I will be stuck on a few numbers that I can never get below. I will be back where I was for years before I started eating healthier; namely, eating less during the week and binging on weekends.

So when I was binging on the weekends I would go from gaining 5 or 6 pounds after the weekend and then back down to my then-goal by the end of the week. I would simply move up and down and never get any lower.

This is why I now weigh myself daily so that I have a lot of data to support and sustain what I am doing. By doing this, I am constantly checking, and the idea is that I am making lifestyle and eating changes so that I am hopefully retraining my body to recognize how much food I actually need, and so that I can become in tune with, and mindful of what it means to be full, and so that I can stop eating when I am full, and not when I am stuffed.

I believe that it is important to have an overall healthy attitude, self-awareness, and self love, for the constant use of the scale as a tool to work in positive ways for me. For example, others with low esteem can be on a emotional roller coaster of self punishment when the scale does not show them what they want to see. So while I am using it as a tool and a guide, others may use it a whipping tool. I acknowledge the need to have self love and patience and note these limitations of the tool and I will talk more about this in chapter 6.

In addition, the way I see it, if I were to still overeat on a few days and "starve" on others, then I am not retraining my body to understand when it is full and I would continue to receive confusing messages.

Calorie Counting

Some weight loss programs require the dieter to calculate calories, or record the foods eaten, or monitor calories burned, and the like. If this is what you are doing and it works for you then by all means keep doing it. To me it just seems too confusing, cumbersome, time consuming, and beside the point. Ultimately, I want to know how much weight I lost, not how many calories I burned, nor how many calories I ate. So it makes sense to me that if my focus is ultimately how much weight I lose, then standing on a scale that measures my weight is the cleanest, simplest, and most accurate way to find that out. And if the number on the scale is larger than I expected, then I simply need to change what I am doing by eating smaller portions, and or eating different types of foods. To me it's very simple and cannot get any simpler.

Or as a dietitian friend of mine said after reading a draft of this book: "Simplest is to eat a high abundance of high nutrient and low calorie foods at every meal i.e. fruits and vegetables."

Counting calories and other approaches is just too complicated for me. To further confuse things, there is even disagreement about how many calories equals a pound. Some say that if you lose 3500 calories then you will lose one pound, and so if you cut 500 calories a day by the end of the week you will lose one pound. Others challenge this calculation and say that it depends on the size of the individual, and how slow or fast their metabolism is and so on. So for me this is all too complicated, and time consuming, and confusing. Keeping it simple worked for me—stand on a scale and modify accordingly. Simple as that. Again, ultimately losing calories is not what I really want to do, but losing body fat is, and so using the measurement of weight rather calories seems to make the most sense to me.

Also, consider this. Again, I am not a calorie expert but this seems to make sense to me. Imagine that you are eating 1000 calories more than what you require to sustain yourself and to be at a healthy weight. Now imagine that you cut 500 calories a day from your diet, in this example, you are still eating 500 calories more than what you need and so you are still not going to lose the weight, but likely continue to gain.

In practice, things may not be so simple. When I asked a dietitian friend of mine if this is the case, she responded with the following: "A person will lose excess body fat even at a 500 calorie reduction due to the un-sustained high calories that support the excessive body fat. This will depend upon the degree of food abuse."

Nevertheless, counting calories might not make this clear, but standing on a scale and looking at your weight certainly will, and standing on a scale will allow you to easily know that you are going to have to eat less or different types of foods to reach your goals. So in my mind there is no need to count calories if you are stepping on the scale daily and using that as your tool. But more importantly than what works for me and what I think, you should embrace whatever works for you.

Also, I am not suggesting that calories are not useful; in fact, I find them to be extremely helpful in determining whether I should eat something and how much of it I should have. My issue is with calorie counting to lose weight and the complexity of that. So before I eat something I do check how many calories it is, and I do find it useful to know whether it is 10 or 1000 calories, and that information I find very useful to help guide me. It really helps me make choices in the moment and for that I am grateful that the number of calories are listed on packages and that the practice is so ubiquitous.

So calories do serve a useful purpose, but sitting there and obsessively counting calories during every meal is too complicated, frustrating, and cumbersome for me. Standing on a scale the next day is much simpler and I can successfully do this without having a clue what the total number of calories I consumed the day before is. I know this because, I have lost the weight by standing on the scale and I have never counted how many calories I consumed in total in a given day. So calories in and of themselves can be important for me, but tallying them up is not very manageable.

Exercise

I often hear, what is more effective for weight loss, exercising or dieting? The consensus on this seems to be clear: If you want to lose weight, eating less and more nutritious foods is the way to do it. Some say that 75% of weight loss is diet related. This makes sense to me, especially when I consider this: I went to an online calculator that estimates the amount of calories burned for certain activities. I tried to stick with the example I used above and so I entered into the website calculator a male who is 5 foot eight and weighs 167 pounds and walks at 4mph (I assume this is a brisk pace because the options were 2, 3, or 4 mph and I chose 4 mph) for 60 minutes will burn 390 calories. In addition, consider this: A small apple with the skin is 53 calories, a 100 g waffle is 291 calories, and two pancakes (232 g) with butter and syrup is 520 calories and so on. It becomes clear, first of all, that having to count calories is a very confusing and time consuming way of losing weight, and second, that depending on what I eat, my calorie count can catch up to me pretty quickly, and so exercising is a very hard way to negate that and to lose weight.

Now I have to say categorically that I am for exercising and I truly believe that exercise is a critical part of healthy living. As my dietitian friend reminded me, "exercise raises a person's metabolic rate and allows for an efficient burning of calories." I exercise every day. In the winter I exercise on my treadmill for one hour every day and in the summer I bike ride every day. In between I also do other things but lately these are my primary forms of exercise. I, however, exercise not to lose weight but because of all of the other health benefits associated with exercising. So, I am in no way urging people not to exercise but simply trying to make the point that exercise is not the primary tool to lose weight, eating less is.

Having said that, I am off on one of my bike rides now. When we were looking for a new home, one condition was that we find a place near where we were so that I could continue to enjoy the benefits of the bike trail near where we lived. There is a river that runs along it and it has both a paved path as well as a dirt path, and it is lined with tress along both sides.

For me biking and exercising is a very holistic experience; it is good for my mind, body, spirit, and emotions. During and after a bike ride my mind feels clear and relaxed. Sometimes when I ride I do so meditatively and sometimes I use my bike ride to help me work through things that I am interested in working through. My body feels great after a bike ride. I feel rejuvenated and I am sure much healthier because of riding. Spiritually I feel open and an overall sense of peace and accomplishment by riding. And emotionally, I feel calm and present. I am very grateful that I incorporate exercising in general and bike riding specifically into my daily routines.

3 WHAT I EAT: MORNING

I often get asked for examples of what types of foods I eat or what does a typical daily food intake look like for me. I think these are great questions and that it is useful to get a sense of what I do so that others can also get a sense and then modify as they see fit. Consequently, in the next 3 sections I will share examples of some meals and portion sizes that work for me. Some of the recipes I played with on my own, some are variations of things I have been eating all of my life, some I adopted after speaking to people and they shared with me their recipes, some I cannot even remember where I got them from, and some resulted from any combination of the above.

This cannot be repeated enough, the way to lose weight is to eat smarter. In this chapter I am going to share with you how changing my eating habits has resulted in my weight loss. To achieve and maintain my long-term-goal I had to do two basic things: I had to eat smarter, first, by eating less, and second, by eating nutritious foods. Fortunately, I am able to eat smarter, in part, because the success I see everyday by standing on the scale helps to keep me motivated and prevents me from lapsing. Because I stand on the scale everyday, I can easily correct what I am doing so that I can easily get back on track if and when the evidence suggests I need to.

Flexibility

Another advantage of this approach to weight loss is in the flexibility it affords. In my mind, this approach transcends culture and preferences. It does not matter if you are a vegan, vegetarian, flexitarian, or meat lover, as long as you watch your portion size and make certain changes to the types of food you eat, this diet can work. It does not discriminate and is very flexible.

In my case I am a vegetarian because I believe that I do not have to kill animals to eat, but if you feel differently this diet will still work for you. So when you read what follows please keep in mind that this is what I did based on my lifestyle and my food preferences, and so feel free to use it if your tastes and ideologies are similar, but if they differ that will not limit your success. The truth is that there are billions of us on this planet and the details and specifics of how each of us will lose weight is as varied as each of us are. Again, as long as I stand on the scale and use it to gather evidence, and I eat less when the evidence suggests I need to, and I make smarter choices, then this weight loss approach works.

Eating Less

I find pictures useful so throughout I am going to share images to help better illustrate how much I eat. In addition, the images will offer a better idea of what the food I eat looks like, in case you want to try some of the recipes that work for me. Note that in the printed version of this book the pictures are in black and white. I decided on this compromise since if the book was printed in color the cost would have practically quadrupled. Given that, I decided that it is best to make the book accessible and affordable so that hopefully more people will benefit.

Breakfast

Let's start with breakfast. It used to be that I would eat a very large portion of a bran based cereal every morning. I find that even too much of a healthy food will result in weight gain. The proof is evident when I stand on the scale, and so through trial and error, like a good researcher, I test what impact eating portions have on my weight. I do not rely on calories or hypothetical scenarios or . . . I simply stand on the scale and that is all the proof I need. It does not matter that it may not make sense in theory; ultimately, the reality is what the reality is. If my weight goes up, then I need to change what I am doing, simple as that.

As I have said throughout, if you are not sure, it is best to consult a professional. For example, my friend who is a dietitian said that, "there are references to serving sizes that provide guidance to people. For example, portions are based on servings. As per the Canada Food Guide, growing people and larger people are advised to eat more servings (larger portions) than smaller and not growing people."

I have been eating bran based cereal for breakfast for most of my life. The problem, I now realize, is that my portion size was enormous in comparison to how much of it I eat now. As an example, I used to buy 4 liters of skim milk every 4 days (and I would be the one in my home consuming most of it); now I find that the expiry date comes and I have to throw out a third of it because it has spoiled. What I use to eat in one sitting will now last me 4 or 5 days. I cut my portion by one-third to one-quarter of what I used to have.

The result is that I feel much better because now I am not bloated after breakfast. I was clearly overestimating how much food I need. When I visit my parents and they are having breakfast, I see where my sense of how much food I thought I needed comes from. Their idea of a portion size, which I have internalized, is enormous. They still have now more than what I used to have. I used to think that I was having a small portion because in comparison to many others around me, my portion was smaller, so I never really thought about how much I was really having versus how much I actually need.

Clearly, my idea of a portion was significantly off. Imagine what would happen if many people started to consume less food, would we have more to go around? Would supply go up and more people be able to afford food? Does the economy need us to overeat and consume more and more? Are people getting rich off of our ill health? Is this sustainable? I find these to be very good and interesting questions, however they seem to be beside the point: The focus of this book is how I can, and by extension, hopefully others, best lose weight and become healthier.

Feel Better

Anyway, clearly I was eating too much and I feel much, much better now that I have brought my portion size in line with what I actually need. My daughters are again great examples for me when it comes to portion size. As I said earlier, we have never force fed them and we allow them to eat when they are hungry and to be free to refuse food without consequences when they are not. This, I believe, has served them well, and has allowed them to listen to and stay in tune with their bodies. They know what it means to be full because their bodies tell them that they are full. As I mentioned above, they are very good about leaving food in their dish when they have had enough, and their portion sizes are not excessive. So as long as they eat the appropriate amount of food, and they look healthy, and they feel healthy, and their medical checkups confirm that, then I can feel confident that they are on a healthy track.

Force-Fed

In contrast, as I said before, when I was a child I was force-fed. I was forced to eat whatever was on my plate and remember, my portion sizes were out of sync with what I actually needed. As a child I was always on the smaller side and so this made things really difficult for me. Sure enough by being force-fed, I learned that being full meant feeling stuffed. I also (mis)learned that the amount of food my body was telling me I needed was not the amount of food I actually needed, and I (mis)learned that what I actually needed was 4 or 5 times more than what my body was telling me. In short, I was trained to overeat and to believe that feeling stuffed is what my body needed to feel satisfied.

Unfortunately, little has changed among many of my circle of friends and family, and as far as I can tell, society at large. I still see infants being overfed. I see infants spitting out food, squirming, struggling to get away, but the adults keep feeding and keep insisting that they are not having enough. The adults truly believe that they know better than the infant what is enough food for them. And the pattern continues all the way through childhood. I see young people of all ages being force-fed, bribed, or punished for not eating what adults think is enough, and the adults never once seem to pause and think that the children are right and they are wrong.

I truly believe that this is why so many of us are so unhealthy, why we have lost touch with our bodies. I believe that force-feeding has broken our ability to self-determine when we are full, and when we should stop eating. I know that when people are doing this, they think that they are helping and improving the others health, unfortunately the result, too often, is that they are doing the exact opposite, they are diminishing people's health.

Here is an image of how much cereal I used to eat versus how much I currently eat. As you can see the difference is huge. What I am having now feels just right and what I used to have was overindulgent.

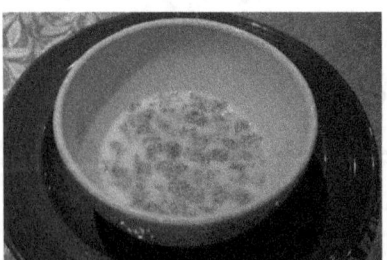 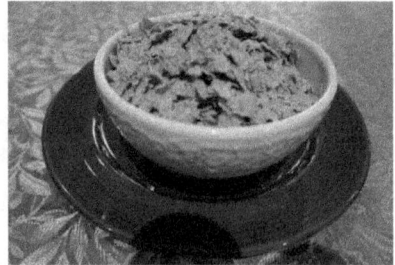

Morning Snack

A few hours after I have my breakfast, I start to feel hungry and so I usually have my morning snack then. The recipe for my morning snack is also something that I played with until I finally found the right recipe for me. My goal is to make a lifestyle change and so I need to enjoy my food, and to make sure that what I have is something I look forward to, and not something that I take just so that I feel full. I think that if I did not enjoy what I was consuming then losing weight would become too much of a chore, and I am not sure I would be able to sustain it the way I now believe I can.

So my morning snack consists of a basic shake. I started out with using skim milk as the base and then decided I could find a better substitute since cholesterol was a concern for me. I tried to substitute skim milk with water but I did not find the taste appealing. Then I tried almond milk and that worked well. It was much tastier for me than water and it improved the taste for me significantly.

When I first started having my shake my portion size was larger than it currently is, and so portion size is another thing that I had to adjust. I started out with a full glass of liquid as a base and I am now down to less than half a glass. Once all the ingredients are added this gives me a large glass full of nutrients. Before I adjusted the portion size to half a glass as my base liquid, I was getting almost two full glasses, which left me feeling stuffed rather than satisfied. I am in a good place now and my body has become used to the amount of food I consume, and I feel satisfied.

So, now my shake consists of just under a half glass of almond milk; half of a banana; half of an apple (I simply place the other halves in a glass container, seal it, place it in the fridge and use it the next day); a packet of maple and brown sugar flavored oatmeal; some frozen or fresh berries (if they are frozen I take them out of the freezer and place what I need in a bowl to thaw; otherwise the shake will be very cold and I prefer it less so); a few dashes of cinnamon; and, more recently, a tablespoon or so full of molasses. I simply place it all in a blender and I liquefy it for about 30 seconds. From time to time I tried to add pieces of kale but I did not find the taste to my liking and so I no longer add it.

As I said previously, this is a lifestyle change and I plan to do this long-term and so I have to enjoy and look forward to what I am consuming. The truth is that I find that, for me, this recipe tastes awesome. I simply love it and I really look forward to having it. I would compare it to a decadent ice-cream shake or a sweet dessert except that it is healthy for me, and what I mean by that is that when I stand on the scale the next day my weight is in check, and if I have ice-cream or a sweet dessert that would definitely not be the case. In short, I love what I am eating and so it does not feel like a sacrifice. I am not sacrificing taste, but just losing weight and that is key for me to sustain my lifestyle changes.

This is a picture of the ingredients I use for my shake as well as what the portion size looks like once blended.

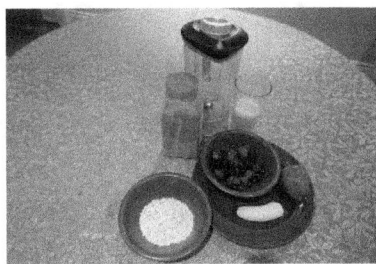 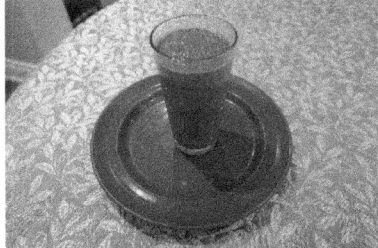

4 WHAT I EAT: LUNCH AND DINNER

In this section I will share a few examples of what I have for lunch and dinner. I have combined lunch and dinner because the truth is that I do not distinguish between lunch meals and dinner meals. Whatever I eat for lunch, I sometimes eat for dinner and vice-versa. In fact, I sometimes do the same for what I have for breakfast, and I have what I have for breakfast as a snack, lunch, or dinner, and the same is true for all of my meals. I usually have the same thing for breakfast and my morning snack because I like what I have and look forward to it so much that if I did not have it, I would miss it. Just a note, that if I have these meals as a snack, my portion is even smaller since it's a snack and I do not need as much to feel satisfied and full.

Lunch And Dinner

Here are some examples of meals that I mostly have for lunch and dinner. I sometimes have a veggie dog with ketchup and a healthy extra thin slice of bread; or 0% fat Greek yogurt with granola and agave nectar; or pasta with sauce and white beans; or a veggie schnitzel with spinach; or eggplant parmesan (I usually buy a premade tray that is a suggested serving size for 4 people and I make at least 8 meals out of it—I freeze the leftover pieces and microwave as needed); or whole wheat penne or spaghetti with sauce and light ricotta cheese; or a grilled veggie cheese sandwich; or tacos with beans and no fat sour cream; or beans; or spelt pasta with ricotta; or a veggie burger with ketchup; or oatmeal; and so on. In case you are interested I will give you a brief description followed by an image to give you a sense of how I prepare each of these meals. The meals are simple and quick to prepare. In some cases I can prepare my meal in mere minutes. It is not meant to be complicated but practical, realistic, and for me, tasty. I have learned that food does not have to be bland to be healthy.

Finally, I see cooking as an art and not a science and so I will not add specific measurements and just urge you to experiment if you are interested in trying any of these recipes. For example, some people like more salt and some less, some like their pasta al dente and others well cooked, and so it's best to play with it and if it suits your taste, then it's right. The idea is to have food that you enjoy, and that is healthy, and that is eaten in small portions because that is all we need.

Veggie Hot Dog

There are a few ways to cook a veggie dog. I have boiled it, baked it in the oven, and placed it on a barbeque. Either way works and which you choose is a matter of personal preference. When I boil it, I simply take a small pot, add water, bring the water to a boil, then add the hotdog for a minute or so. It does not take very long at all to cook. Rather than using a hotdog bun, I then take a slice of healthy toast bread and place the hotdog in, add ketchup, and sometimes sliced pickles, and eat it. It is quick, simple, tasty, and very healthy. As you introduce various meals you can see the impact it has by simply standing on the scale the next day and using it as a tool so that you know if your portion and the type of foods you are eating results in achieving the goal you set.

The pictures I am sharing are not meant to be professional shots, but it is a realistic look at the foods I am actually eating. I have never taken a course on food preparation or photography. I am not trying to stage things, but I am simply capturing what I am actually about to eat. It is not meant to entice, but to inform, and share.

Below is a picture of a veggie dog, a slice of healthy bread, and ketchup. For this meal I also had roasted eggplant and zucchini on the side.

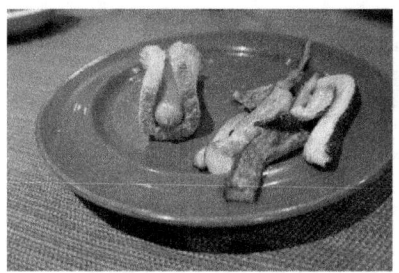

0% Fat Greek Yogurt With Granola And Agave Nectar

This is great as lunch, dinner, a snack, or even as dessert. When I started experimenting with this recipe, I found it was too bland and therefore I was not enjoying it. I knew that I had to play with the recipe. I then decided to add sugar and that worked, it was delicious, but I found that it did not sit well with me. I then decided to substitute the sugar with agave nectar and that made the recipe both delicious and my body seemed to respond better to the agave than the sugar and so that is what I stick with.

So now I have about a tablespoon or a tablespoon and a half of the yogurt, I sprinkle some granola on top (not too much but enough), mix it, and then I drizzle very small amounts of agave nectar. As I eat it and when the agave is gone from inside the bowl, I drizzle a little more, again being very conscious not to add too much.

Below is a picture of my bowl of 0% fat Greek yogurt with granola and agave nectar.

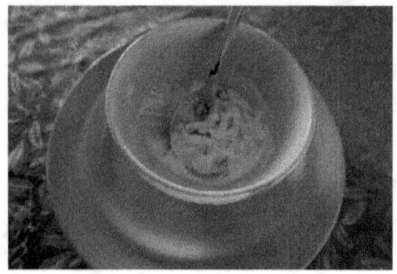

Pasta With Sauce And White Beans (if desired you can add light ricotta and or spinach)

This is a very delicious dish. I find it to be healthy and delicious. This can take a little more time, but not much. The taste is worth it. I simply boil water in a medium size pot. I add salt to the water. Then once it boils I usually add whole wheat tubetti pasta (you can also use white pasta, or elbow pasta or whatever your heart desires really). With all of these recipes feel free to play and experiment until you find what works best for you. When the pasta is halfway cooked, I open a can of white beans and add them to the pot. Once the pasta is cooked, I drain most of the water and add a small amount of sauce. How much is also based on preference. For example, I like adding a little more sauce and my daughter prefers a little less. At this point I sometimes add some spinach and let it cook with the spinach in the pot for a few minutes. Then once it's cooked to how I like it, I simply put it in a plate, and add light ricotta on top (or even parmesan cheese if you prefer). Before I started my lifestyle change I use to eat at least two hearty plates of the pasta, I now have about a quarter of one plate and it satisfies me.

Below is a picture of my serving of pasta with sauce, white beans, spinach, and light ricotta on top.

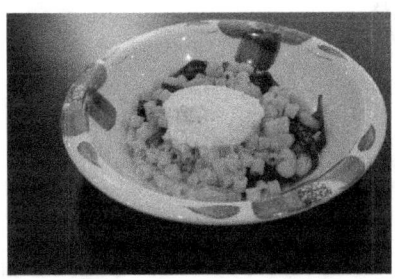

Veggie Schnitzel With Spinach

This is also very tasty for me. I bake the schnitzel in the oven and while it is cooking I prepare the spinach. To prepare the spinach, I get two pans and I turn one upside down and place it over the other and use it as a lid. I put the oven burner very, very low and I add spinach to the pan and nothing else. I then place the other pan that I am using as a lid on top and I stir it periodically. Once the schnitzel is ready I take it out of the oven and place it on a dish. I then take the spinach and usually place it on top of the schnitzel. At this point I add salt to the spinach and I eat it. All of these dishes seem to react well with my body and help keep my weight in check. Finding what I like and what works is key to a healthy diet.

Below is a picture of my veggie schnitzel with spinach on the side.

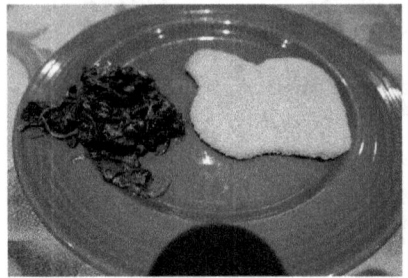

Eggplant Parmesan

I am adding this because it is something that I truly enjoy and it is very simple to make. I also wanted to share an example of how prepared meals are also an option. Everything need not be made from scratch. I buy a tray of this at a local Italian catering place for $9.99. It comes in various sizes and it is very reasonably priced. It's like lasagna (which more people might be familiar with), except instead of noodles, slices of eggplant is used in its place. I simply cut it into serving sized pieces, and put some in the fridge because I know I will consume it over the next few days, and I put the rest in a container and place it in the freezer for later use. To heat it, I simply place it on a flat dish and I add a pasta dish or deeper bowl on top to cover it so that the sauce and contents of the eggplant does not splat all over the microwave as it heats up. I set the timer, and about 40 seconds later, it is ready to eat. Fast, delicious, and healthy.

This is a fairly inexpensive meal especially since a serving tray of 4 portion sizes, is really a portion size of 8 for me. Another way that places make money is that they underestimate the portion sizes. This might also be done because, as the saying goes, it is better to have more than not enough, and especially when I am hosting people I can see that pressure playing itself out. Recently we had guests over and they had just thrown a party for 25 guests. They ordered food from a catering service for 25 and they said all they really needed to order was food for 15, since they had so much left over. Having said that, were they to do it again, they will still order for 25 even though 15 was plenty, admittedly, as would I, which I am sure would please any caterer.

Below is a picture of the eggplant parmesan in a tray, and then a portion size in my dish with baked peas and mushrooms, and green beans on the side.

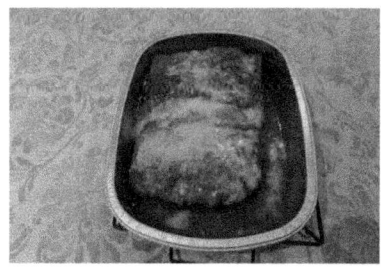 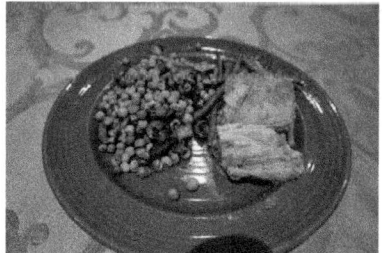

Whole Wheat Penne Or Spaghetti With Sauce, Basil And Light Ricotta Cheese

This is yet another simple and delicious recipe. Making pasta is simple and fairly quick. Once a year we get together with several families and we make our own home-made sauce, place it in jars, and use it as needed. But store bought sauce jars also work well. To make the pasta I simply boil water, and add salt. Once the water boils, I add the pasta. Once it's cooked, I pour the contents in a colander to drain the water. Then I pour the pasta back into the pot, and add a little sauce. Then I mix the pasta and sauce by stirring it. I then put the pasta in plates and add more sauce if and as desired. Finally, I add a spoon full of light ricotta cheese on top, if desired. If I am making the spaghetti, the process is exactly the same, just instead of boiling the penne I boil spaghetti or whatever other type of pasta I prefer. Also, I sometimes add an assortment of vegetables to the mix. For example, I sometimes add peppers, mushrooms, broccoli and so on, to the sauce. This makes it both flavorful and nutritious.

Below is a picture of penne with sauce, basil leaves, and light ricotta; and a picture of spaghetti with sauce, and parmesan cheese on top.

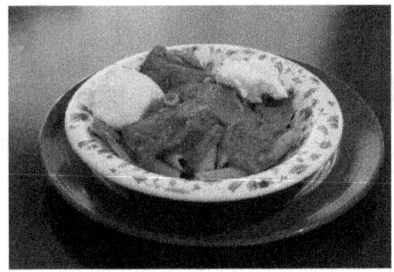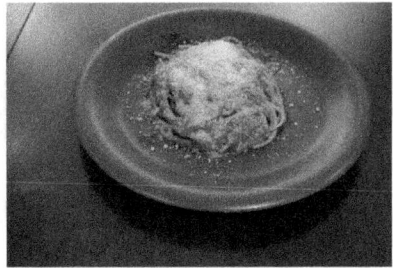

Grilled Veggie Cheese Sandwich

For this I use thin sliced healthy whole wheat toast bread. I lightly butter a slice of bread and then place it in a pan butter side down. The pan is somewhat hot, since I heat in on low for a minute or so. The key to this for me is that the burner needs to be on low and the pan needs to have a lid placed on top of it to help hold in the heat and melt the veggie cheese. I then place a slice of veggie cheese on the bread that is in the pan. Then I very lightly butter another slice of bread and place it butter side up over the bread and cheese that is in the pan. I then place a lid on the pan and let in sit for awhile. The way I do it the burner is on low because I prefer my grilled veggie cheese sandwich to not be crisp, so cooking it takes some time. I then flip the sandwich and wait for it to cook. Once it's done it's ready to eat. I like my sandwich very soft and squishy, others I know prefer it darker, and so cook to whatever your preference is.

Below is a picture of my grilled cheese sandwich.

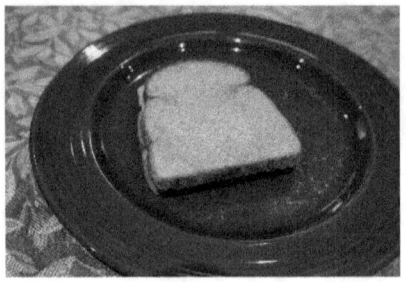

Tacos With Beans And No Fat Sour Cream

For this recipe I use a can of red beans and another of black beans. First, I rinse the beans in a colander. Then, I simply add water to a pan, and add a package of taco mix, and the beans. I then cook it until most of the water is dried up. Once it's ready I place it in tacos, add some no fat sour cream and eat it. I sometimes add diced tomatoes and lettuce.

Below is a picture of tacos with beans, lettuce, tomatoes, and no fat sour cream.

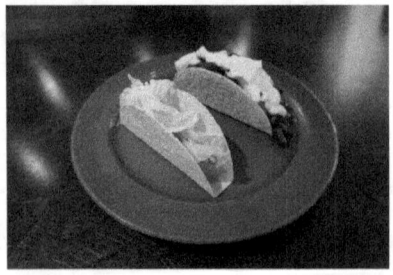

Beans And Peas

White Beans

Beans and peas make for a very healthy meal and depending

on what type of beans I am eating, I either have it cold or hot. For example, if I am having white beans, first, I rinse the beans in a colander. Then I simply add water to a pot, add the beans, salt, and oil and then place the pot on the stove. Once it boils I drain the water, add oregano, and they are ready to eat.

Below is a picture of white beans.

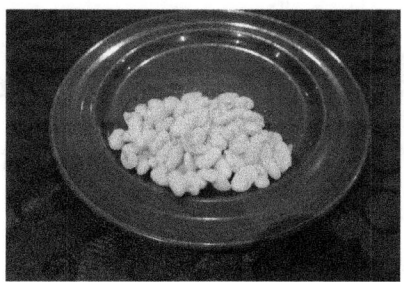

Black-Eyed Peas

If I am having black-eyed peas, I make bean soup with it. First, I rinse the beans in a colander. Then I simply open the can, place the beans in a pot, add water, salt, and oil. Once it comes to a boil, I eat it as a soup.

Below is a picture of my black-eye pea soup.

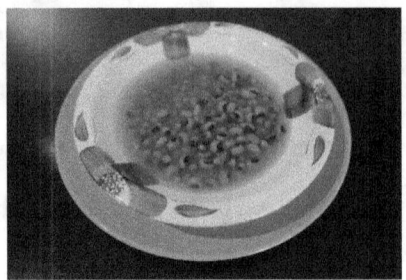

Red Beans, Bean Medley, Chic Peas

If I am having red beans, bean medley, or chic peas I simply open the can, rinse the beans in a strainer, make sure all the water is drained, place it in a small bowl, add salt, and oil, and eat it as a cold salad.

Below is a picture of red beans, bean medley, and chic peas.

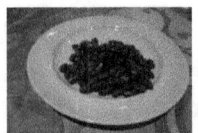 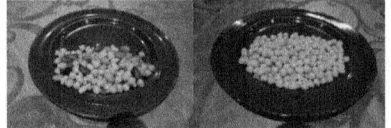

Black Beans

If I am making black beans, I wash the beans in a strainer, place them in a bowl or on a plate, add oil, and salt and place it in the microwave for about 45 seconds and I eat it that way.

Below is a picture of my black beans.

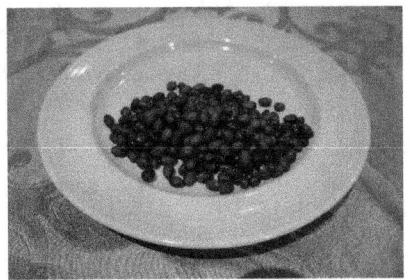

Even too much of a good thing can be too much and overindulgent. However I have my beans, I always remember to have a small portion. I usually, make just as much as I am going to eat and then I place the rest in a container and store it in the fridge and use it for another meal.

Spelt Pasta With Light Ricotta

This is a recipe that my wife makes. I really enjoy eating it. She simply boils water, adds oil, salt, and the spelt pasta. Once it's cooked, she adds the light ricotta and I eat it like a soup.

Below is a picture of my spelt pasta with light ricotta.

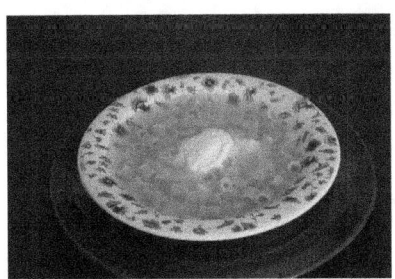

Veggie Pattie/Burger With Ketchup

I usually place my veggie burger in the oven and once it's

cooked I put it on a plate, add ketchup, and eat it. I sometimes will have corn, or eggplant, or peppers, or mushrooms and peas baked in the oven and eat those with my veggie burger or pattie.

Below is a picture of my veggie pattie with corn and spinach on the side.

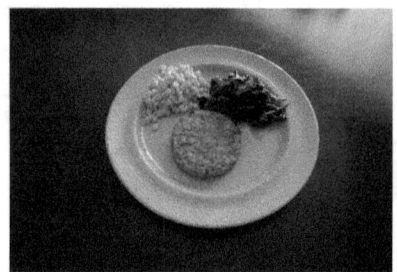

Oatmeal

For my oatmeal I have had to experiment to find a recipe that tastes best to me and that is healthy. At first, I would simply put milk in a bowl, add plain quick oats and have it as is. Truthfully, for me the taste was too bland and if I am going to make this change I want to make sure that I am enjoying my food. I then tried to add brown sugar and that made it tasty but too decadent. I then tried to add some maple syrup and that also did not work for me. I liked the taste but when I weighed myself on the scale the next day, I was not happy with the number and so I continued to modify until I found both what tastes good and what does not impact my weight.

So what I do now is that I take skim milk and place it in a

bowl, I then add a packet of oatmeal (maple and brown sugar) to the bowl, and then I add some more plain quick oats to make it a more filling portion for me. This combination is perfect for me: it fills me up, has the right amount of sweetness that makes it really tasty for me, and it allows me to reach and maintain my long-term weight goal.

Below is a picture of my oatmeal in a bowl.

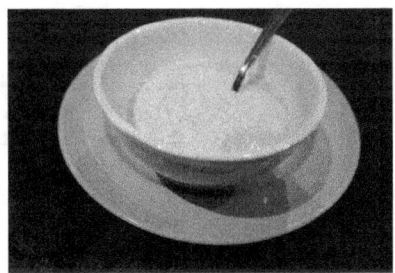

Tinkering

Eating right and figuring out what works for me is not difficult, but it does require some tinkering as I figure out exactly what works for me. For me the results are what keep me motivated. The data and the evidence helps me maintain the will required to continue to eat well. Being disciplined is not easy, but it requires just that: discipline. If I want to lose weight and get healthier bad enough, then I need to do what I need to do to reach my long term goal.

5 WHAT I EAT: SNACKS AND DESSERT

Like many people, I love sweets and so if I am going to make this work I need to find a way to fit some type of sweets in my diet. Fortunately, there are plenty of options and some have much less of an impact on my weight than others. I quickly discovered that rather than having a piece of cake or ice-cream or some other high calorie, high fat dessert, I can have sweets that will have much less of an impact on my weight and that will allow me to achieve my long-term goal. The same applies to what I eat as snacks in-between meals. I need to continue to watch portion sizes and make smarter choices. Again, fortunately there are plenty of tasty yet healthier options that work for me given my goal.

Snacks

Some of the snacks that I find work well for me are dried chickpeas, nuts, carrots, lupini, pickles, peaches, plums, cantaloupe, melon, cherries, and other fruits and vegetables. It is necessary for me to keep in mind that if I want to reach my goal, simply because they are healthier options does not mean that I can eat an unlimited amount. I often hear people say that you can eat all of the fruits and vegetables that you want. For me, this is not the case. I know that I cannot because when I step on the scale the next morning, the number on the scale alerts me that I need to modify what I am doing if I want to reach my goal. In addition, there is no need for me to overeat on fruits and vegetables because once I am full, there is no need to eat more. I do not have to reach the point of feeling stuffed to be satisfied. Also, if I know that I have eaten enough and my body is telling me that I need more, then I simply walk away because my body could be wrong. At that point, I have to make a decision based on whether I have had enough food to eat, and if I know that I have then I will feel that I have made the correct decision.

This is why I often hear people say that before you have dessert walk away, and then you will find that more often than not you will no longer want to have it. This is because it takes awhile for our bodies to register that we are full. I appreciate this advice, and the fact that after I walk away I no longer want it, is a testament that I did not need it in the first place. As time goes on and my body is retrained, I find that I am better (not perfect) at being able to keep to smaller portions and smarter food choices. As I have said before, rather than placing large amounts on my plate, I just put a small amount and I find that more often than not, that is more than enough. I have come to know how much food I need and I am better at putting a smaller portion on my plate than having a larger portion and leaving left overs once I am full. If I put a larger portion, even if I tell myself that I will leave some on my plate, inevitably I will overeat. Again, I am not perfect and I need strategies and putting small portions on my plate is one that really works for me. After I eat it, I am full and fine with the serving size. Having said that, I am learning to leave food on my plate when I feel that I am full.

Snacks are useful ways of giving me the nutrition I need and of assuring me that I am getting the right amount of food. Snacking helps ensure that I do not feel very hungry, by giving me just the right amount in between my larger meals. Interestingly, before I started eating healthier, if I waited too long to eat, predictably I would get a headache that would only go away by me sleeping it off. This is no longer the case. I can go a longer time without food and it no longer results in headaches. I am not sure why this is or what it means, but it is something that I noticed. Having said that, I am really good at eating frequently and very rarely am I in a situation where I go long stretches without food.

Snacks are definitely important, but they too need to be consumed in small portions. So if I have carrot sticks as a snack, then I only have about one sliced carrot or less depending on my need. I find what helps is to have these healthy snacks easily available. I usually cut them in advance and place them in a container in the refrigerator, that way when I am ready for a snack it is easy to access and consume.

If I have corn on the cob as a snack, I will have 1 or 2 pieces. If I have pickles, I will have 2 or 3. If I have lupini beans, I will have 10 or 12. If I have nuts, I will have 3 pistachios; or 3 pieces of walnut; or 3 almonds; or 2 cashews; or a small handful of sunflower or pumpkin seeds. I know my body needs food and variety and so I make sure it gets it. I also know that I need nowhere near the enormous amounts of foods our society has made us believe we need, or the amount I once thought I needed.

In addition, we might want to eat so much because we can afford it and like the taste. I think it is much more complicated and that, in part, we also over consume for reasons beyond what advertising says.

The food I now eat is always a small portion because that is all I need. I purposely use the word "I" throughout this book as much as possible because this is what I do and what I have found works for me. You might find that different approaches work for you. The one constant is that when you stand on the scale the next day, you will get all of the feedback you need, and your limits may very well be different than mine. Your body and metabolism might react different to the portion sizes and types of foods than does mine, and if you are reaching the goal you set while still eating smarter and becoming healthier then you can be assured that what you are doing is right for you.

Below is a picture of lupine and a plate with walnuts, pumpkin seeds, sunflower seeds, cashews, almonds, and pistachios. In fact this is my daily morning snack that I have sometime after my morning cereal and before my morning shake.

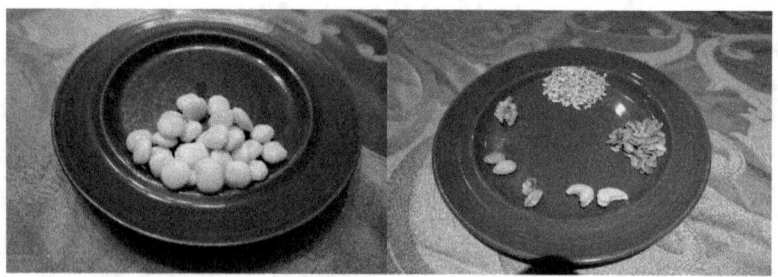

Dessert

I have discovered that changing my lifestyle does not mean that I cannot have dessert, but what it does mean is that I can still have dessert or sweets as long as I continue to eat smarter, and let the scale be my tool. Rather than eating cookies, and cakes, and ice-cream and other high-calorie, high-fat options, I now eat candy (I know that eating candy might not fit my definition of nutritious foods, but to me it is smarter than the more decadent options); and apple slices with cinnamon and sugar; and fruits; and yogurt with granola and agave; and herbal tea with molasses, and honey, or agave instead; and so on.

Having tea is often just as satisfying as having a piece of the dessert, the sweetness is fulfilling and the bonus is that it is healthier. Having tea works well for me as a substitute for dessert. I find that eating smarter choices helps keep me on track, and that I do not miss having the other more overindulgent choices.

Having said that, does this mean I will never have any of those more overindulgent foods again? Clearly not. Since changing my lifestyle, I have very occasionally consumed foods that I know will change the scale, but when I have, I do so in such moderation that it has had little impact on my short-term goal, even less on my milestones, and no impact on my long-term goal. The example, I offer below will make what I mean clearer.

Staying on track can be more challenging when my wife and children and I have dinner plans with friends or other family, especially when the plans are on consecutive days. For example, recently we were invited for dinner on three consecutive days and I used various strategies to help me stay on track. Doing so allowed me to enjoy being with people, partake in the feast while not overeating, tasting the dessert that I desired, all while staying on track in the short-term and the longer-term.

For the first dinner, I knew the people well enough that I shared that I was in the midst of a lifestyle change and explained to them that if I am not being my usually overindulgent self, this is why. Of course, everyone is always very supportive and understanding. I also felt comfortable enough to bring some candy for everyone to share, and this way if I felt the need for something sweet I knew that there would surely be something that I could have and that would not impact my goal. Another good idea is to bring fruit that I like and that are a treat, maybe the first batch of cherries for the season. Anyway, by bringing candy, I was able to mostly eat accordingly. Also important was for me to stay within my portion size, and I mostly did. The next day when I stood on the scale I was slightly off, but not surprised, or worried. I knew that I would simply need to adjust, and I did.

So when we went out on the second outing for dinner at another of our friends' place, I was more careful and also shared with them in advance what I was doing so that they would not go to extra trouble, and that they would know in advance that I would be eating smarter. I also brought candy there and it worked well. By the next day when I stood on the scale, I started to veer back on track.

The third day, it was a larger gathering and so I did not feel I had to make them aware that I would be eating little. I did not know them as well and did not feel it was appropriate to bring candy. We were asked to bring things and so we made sure to bring things that I felt was healthy and if there was nothing else that I wanted, I would be able to have what we contributed to the potluck. Of course there was plenty of food and I was able to pick and choose and had a great meal that was well within my portion size.

Come dessert everyone was raving and so rather than avoid dessert altogether, I simply took very, very small portions of two out of the three desserts offered, and the next day I was still on track. For one dessert I had about a small fork full. When I say small, I mean small. It looked good but the other was my preference, so I decided to have just enough to try it. It was one bite, and I tried it, and it was good, and I was satisfied that I had tried it. The other dessert I had a little more of but still a sliver. So rather than inhaling it or ravaging it like a vulture consuming a carcass, I decided to savor it. I decided to have a small morsel and to enjoy each and every bite. After all, I was having it not because I was hungry, because I was not, but simply because it was delicious and dessert, and because it was there and everyone else was having some. In short, I was able to taste the dessert and so not miss out while staying on track.

I share these stories as a way of trying to offer a sense of how I deal with real-life scenarios, hopefully, in the process painting a clearer picture of how I have made it work.

When I first started to eat smarter and healthier, I knew that my biggest tests would come during parties and functions, and that has proven to be the case. The first few times were much more difficult than it is now, although I still have the odd lapse. I think I needed to figure out if I could indeed resist and eat less when in the company of others, and with more food that was sitting there tempting me to indulge.

To date I have been able to do so very successfully. In fact, there has only been one occasion near the beginning of my journey where I did overeat. The next day when I stepped on the scale I was able to see the results that such a binge would have. I did not beat myself up but simply got back on track, and that took a number of days to do. Maybe because I did see the impact of overeating on my goal, I have not deviated in that way since.

Apple, Cinnamon, and Sugar

One dessert that really satisfies my cravings for sweets and seems to agree with me is apple, cinnamon, and sugar. I take an apple slicer and cut the apple in slices. Then I take a container that has a lid, and I add sugar, and very little cinnamon (when my daughters have it, they add a lot more cinnamon and so it comes down to personal taste). I then place the lid on the container and shake the cinnamon and sugar to mix them together. Finally, I place a few slices of apple at a time in the container and I shake the container. The sugar and cinnamon sticks to the sides of the apple and it tastes really delicious. I have learned now that one apple actually is too much for me, and so I place the extra slices in the fridge and save them for another time. Sometimes they slightly brown but that does not bother me. I sometimes have this as a snack and sometimes as a dessert.

Below is a picture of a slice of apple covered in cinnamon and sugar.

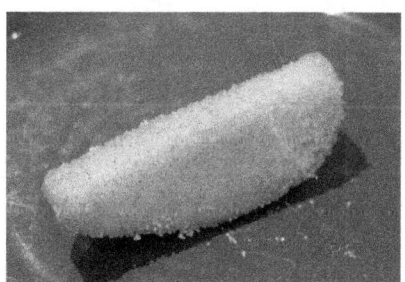

What I Eat In A Typical Day

Since many ask me what I eat in a typical day, here is an example that hopefully you will find worthwhile as I continue to try and share with you what I am doing to become healthier. So here is what a typical day's worth of meals look like for me. This is typical and what I actually ate on Monday, May 25, 2015. For breakfast at 7:30 a.m. I had my bran based cereal. At around 8:30 a.m. I had a mixture of nuts and seeds (2 cashews, 2 almonds, 2 pistachios, 2 pieces of walnut, some plain sunflower seeds without salt and oil, and some plain pumpkin seeds). For my mid-morning snack at 9:50 a.m. I had my shake. For lunch at 11:50 a.m. I had yogurt with granola and agave. As a snack at 1:50 p.m. I had 2 pickles, and at 2:50 p.m., I had 12 cherries. For dinner at 3:45 p.m. (I'll say more about my early dinner routine later) I had whole-wheat penne with sauce, basil, and ricotta. I also had a few pieces of candy after dinner.

Hopefully this gives you a good sense of what and when I eat. Some days I have a few more small snacks, but this is a good indication of a typical day for me.

The table below is a visual of what I describe above, and that I ate Monday, May 25, 2015.

Breakfast at 7:30 a.m.	Bran based cereal
Morning snack at 8:30 a.m.	Mixture of nuts and seeds (2 cashews, 2 almonds, 2 pistachios, 2 pieces of walnut, some plain sunflower seeds

	without salt and oil, and some plain pumpkin seeds).
Mid-morning snack at 9:50 a.m.	Shake with fruit, almond milk, cinnamon, flaxseed, molasses, and an maple oatmeal packet
Lunch at 11:50 a.m.	Yogurt with granola and agave
Snack at 1:50 p.m.	2 pickles
Snack at 2:50 p.m.	I had 12 cherries
Dinner at 3:45 p.m.	Whole-wheat penne with sauce, basil, and ricotta

Good Food Is Good Food

Again, I do not make a huge distinction between any of the categories, but have what I want despite whether it is lunch, dinner, snack, or dessert. I think since I am eating smarter, most of what I eat is a healthy choice and it is never a problem to eat something that is healthy. Eating smarter and healthy does not mean food has to be bland or distasteful, and I recognize that now, which makes things easier. The key is portion size and so whether I am having candy or apples, I always eat very small portions. If I am not sure how much is too much, the scale will tell me. Usually, a couple of pieces is enough to satisfy the sweet craving, there is never a need to overeat no matter how much I might want to.

6 WHAT DO LOVE, TRUST, RESPECT, CARE, AND COMPASSION HAVE TO DO WITH DIETING?

In another book titled, *The Willed Curriculum, Unschooling, and Self-Direction: What Do Love, Trust, Respect, Care, and Compassion Have to do with Learning?* I write about how we learn best when we are in a loving environment and we love what we do. We learn best when we trust ourselves and others trust that what we are learning is worthwhile for us, and that we are supported to continue to pursue our passions. We learn best, when we are respected enough to be supported to learn what we want rather than having someone else tell us what to learn, when, how, where, and why. And of course, we learn best, when we are in a caring and compassionate space and place, and when we become caring and compassionate to ourselves, others, all beings in the world, and the world itself.

In this chapter I would like to extend that argument and apply it to the theme of this book. So what do love, trust, respect, care, and compassion have to do with becoming healthy?

Love

In terms of love, if I love myself and all beings and things within the world, then it would make sense that I would want to become healthy so that I can become the best person I can be. Being as healthy as I can, will also place me in the best position mentally, physically, spiritually, and emotionally to serve myself and all beings and things in the universe.

I believe that love is the driving force to a better me and a better world. Love is what inspires me to try and do the right things. Of course, being human, like everyone else I have lapses. I do things that I wish I did not, but rather than beating myself up, I try to make amends, and if it's not possible, I try to do better the next time. In addition, I think about what I did and when the same situation arises on another occasion, I try and use my experience to do better, rather than simply keep making the same mistakes.

Furthermore, the more I love myself, it makes sense that the healthier I should want to be, and part of good health is loving ourselves. This has nothing to do with narcissism but is connected to having respect for ourselves. Enough respect that

I will allow love to be my guide, and if I love myself, I want what is best, and I want to take care of myself. And as I said earlier, the better I take care of myself, the better position I am in to take care of others. Love is not about imposing, and forcing, and insisting, but it is about trusting, and respecting, and caring. By loving someone I cannot force them to do what I believe to be right, but I can only love them unconditionally and hope that by loving them they will feel the love and in turn will love themselves enough to make positive changes.

Of course, there is no one way to live and to act in a right way, and so respecting diversity and loving unconditionally is key and the essence of love. I believe in freedom, and democracy, and community. All of these things can co-exist and they are not mutually exclusive. I believe that holistically all of this is interconnected. We all have a worldview and a part of good health is to have an open and respectful worldview.

Trust

In terms of trust we need to create spaces and places where people can trust themselves and learn to trust others. In many cases my body has led me astray and I have to work to get it back to the point where I can trust it again, back to the point where I can trust what it is telling me. Where I can trust that when it signals me that it is hungry, that it is indeed hungry and not just addicted or being overindulgent. As I have argued all along, what my body needs is no where near what it wants. I needed to recognize that what it wants is making me unhealthy and that I have to work holistically with my body and get back in tune with what it needs.

I need to trust that I can get there again. I need to trust that my body can be fixed and that it can learn to signal what it needs when it needs it, and I need to listen. I need to listen intently to what my body is telling me, and I need to understand the difference between when it tells me it needs something versus when it tells me it wants what it does not need. Again, I do not believe that I have to be an ascetic to be this person. I can still very much enjoy life and enjoy food, but in order to do that I do not have to overeat.

Respect

Having respect for myself and for others is a central part of creating and living a healthy lifestyle. If I respect myself, then I will live in a certain respectful way. And if I respect other beings and other things in the world, then I will want to take and use only what I need rather than to overeat. If I respect my mind, body, spirit, and emotion I will treat them in a certain way.

To me respect is a part of why I have decided to be a vegetarian. I know others do not see it this way, and that they have a very different definition of respect, and I am open to accepting that. Of course, I still hope that more people will be convinced that they do not have to kill to eat, but all I can do is live my life my way, and then hope that others might also see it the same way. I do not look down on those who disagree with me, but continue to live and walk with my head raised high and understand that others will do the same. I am always open to sharing my message, but never to impose it. I try to live my life humbly and openly and I fully recognize that others have different definitions of what even those terms mean.

Care And Compassion

Ultimately, I see care and compassion as something that I have to continue to strive for. I need to care and show compassion to myself and to others. When I do good I have to recognize that, when I have lapses I have to have care and compassion for myself and for the being or things that I have wronged. There is no end, but this is a continuous process and I believe that healthy living requires that love, respect, trust, care, and compassion all play a central role.

After reading a draft of my book here are some comments that a friend of mine made. I feel that reproducing his comments here and sharing another's story is a good way to end this chapter. This is what he wrote:

"I have had some real success in the past with weight loss. I dropped 100 pounds when I went to university. It took me two years, and, like you I religiously weighed myself each morning and kept that cardinal number in mind all day while I made food choices. Also like you, I had many people ask me for my 'secret,' but I think they didn't really listen to my advice because it didn't involve a gimmick or easy shortcut. I kept that weight off for about 15 years. I've gained weight off and on for the past ten years. I have no real excuse, but I know that when my life was less stressful (especially before having kids) I seemed to have an easier time focusing on my eating habits; I was almost fanatical."

"As I mentioned in an earlier email, I have lost 30 pounds since August 9, 2014 when I bought my new digital scale (I was moved by a number of things, including my brother-in-law who had just noticeably lost weight). Smaller portions have always helped me. I was in the hospital once when I was in first year university with an asthma attack and I was shocked at the portions I was given. They would give you almost anything, but in sensible portions. It was an eye-opener."

"In my own experience, I learned that most people allow (or use) a minor slip in their regimen to completely derail their plan. I found that as long as I was consistently following my plan most of the time, I could still lose weight, even if I occasionally (inconsistently) 'fell off the horse.' As you wrote, soon enough the scale would show that I had weathered the mistake and got back on the horse. In other words, failure is no excuse to stop trying to succeed!"

"Also, as I implied in my narrative above, there is an inescapable psychological dimension to weight loss that can sometimes, for some people, thwart even the most rigorously thought-out plan. For others, discipline comes easier. Many people know what to do, but doing it is another thing. I quit smoking during my first year of university; I found it fairly easy to do, but then again, I had the luxury of simply never again putting another cigarette in my mouth and lighting it. We cannot quit food 'cold turkey.' I see successful weight loss as being truly holistic in the sense that it is a discipline of mind and body. I have heard it said that obesity is a disease of disappointment. Hunger has many sources, and I believe that some of us are starved in our mind, rather than our body."

I appreciate his narrative for adding to the grander story of challenges, struggles, and successes. The journey to better health can be challenging, but if we will it, it can happen. In reading his account, my dietitian friend questioned his use of the word failure and raised a good point. She said, "the word failure is harsh. It is normal to rise and fall with enthusiasm until the way of less eating becomes normal and desirable."

7 CONCLUSION

Living a healthy lifestyle is not easy. Unfortunately, I know far too many people who want to lose weight, have tried, and failed. I am hoping that this book will help many to understand that they can muster their will and live healthier. When I first starting thinking about making changes I was not sure whether I could do it, but now I truly feel that I can sustain the changes I have made. Of course, only time will tell, but at this point I feel that I am passed the hump, and that I have found a lifestyle change that is positive for me and that works. I was always very good at maintaining a certain weight, albeit not in the healthiest way, but I never really tried to seriously lose weight until now. So far I am pleased with how it has gone and I am hoping that my experience will help others who have a similar wish.

Society And Portion Sizes

I find that society at large is not very supportive of people who watch their portion sizes. Society seems to model that we need to consume and spend more and more, and eat more and more, not less. When my family and I go out to dinner we often skip appetizers and share a meal. This is not out of cheapness, which some might assume, but because our idea of a portion size is out of whack with what almost all establishments believe a portion size to be. I find myself feeling guilty or out of place for not conforming, and I often ask myself why do I feel this way? Why am I the strange one for sharing a meal, and others who eat four times what a portion size should be, are normal? I try to compensate by offering a larger tip so that they see that it is not the money that I am concerned about, but that it is simply too much food. Also, whether we are treated to a meal by others, or we are treating others to a meal we still order the same way, so whether we are paying or not is not the point, better health is. Same applies when I am at an all-you-can-eat buffet, I still eat the smarter way.

No Rigid Rules

Another strategy that I have yet to mention is that I almost always eat nothing after 4 p.m., which is when we have dinner as a family. Of course, if I am going out and having dinner somewhere else or if someone is coming over to our house for dinner, I make exceptions. The rules are never rigid but always flexible, and the scale is my tool.

I need to mention that eating after 4 p.m. is nothing new for me. I have been doing it for 20 years and so I do not see this as a significant part of my new approach to becoming healthier. Having said that, I believe it does help to keep my food intake in check since I know that I am not going to eat during such a large part of my waking day.

Water

I also almost always drink just water and never alcohol. I simply do not like the taste of alcohol and so I do not have it. Other drinks I find are simply not worth the calories, and I would rather use the calories for more nutritious things than pop or other less healthy drink options.

Balance Between Mind, Body, Spirit, And Emotions

I believe that the key is for me to listen to my mind and not always rely on my body because I have learned through experience that my body cannot always be trusted. Of course, as holistic beings living in a holistic world we have many faculties that are interconnected and we need to rely on them all in trying to determine what is best. Sometimes my body might fail, but I can then use my other faculties to confirm that I am making the correct choice, and sometimes my body might need to confirm what my mind is telling me. We are complicated beings. Even after my body becomes more in tune, I need to check and make sure that what it is signaling makes sense.

I was so used to listening to someone else tell me what a

portion size is that I lost my ability to gauge for myself. I am not sure I will ever fully get that ability back, and so using my mind and even an external tool like the scale I find to be necessary. Here I agree with a friend who said to me, "I think of the scale as a tool, and my body, mind, emotions, and spirit as the guide." I can easily be deceived and tempted by the delicious taste of food that it is easy to give in, and so attention is required from me. I need to remain vigilant and mindful to ensure I remain as healthy as I can.

The idea is not to starve myself to weight loss, but to become healthier. So I need to make sure that I eat enough, while recognizing the problem, which is that mostly what I believed to be a portion size is way, way too much.

If you are unsure it is always best to check with a professional to ensure that what you are doing is getting healthier rather than less healthy. We all have different body types and there is variability in how much we need to eat to sustain ourselves, and what our ideal weight should be.

For me I had to cut my portion size to a third and even to a quarter of what I used to eat. As I write this I just finished a meal where I had pasta with beans and spinach and ricotta. My daughter prefers it without the spinach and so I took hers out of the pot before I added the spinach to mine. What I left in the pot and thought would be a good portion size for me ended up being two servings. Had I put it all on my plate I would likely have had a hard time not eating it all. Not because I am hungry, but just because it is there. So I simply put on my plate a portion size. Although, as I said earlier, I am getting better at leaving things on my plate when I feel full.

Only Put What You Need On The Plate

I am glad I did what I learned to do, which is to put on my plate only what I have come to know to be a portion size for me. In this case, what I put on my plate proved to be more than enough, and in fact if there was less in my plate I would have also been satisfied. I was recently at a relatives house for lunch and they gave me a large portion and asked me to just eat what I wanted. I know from experience that this will inevitably result in me overeating and so I re-portioned my size and I was glad that I did. I ate what was in my plate and that was more than enough.

If I stand on the scale on one day and I find that I am off track, then I simply get myself back on track the next. Weighing myself everyday allows me to quickly respond and make corrections.

Again, since I have been trained to eat everything on my plate and I find it hard to condition myself to do otherwise, what I find works well is to simply make less and have less on my plate, much, much less than what I was used to. What does not always work for me is to put lots on my plate and then to eat just as much as I need. I find that even now if I have lots on my plate I am tempted to overeat, and so the best thing for me to do is to put a realistic portion size on my plate and I find that it is enough.

I am still getting used to how little I actually need to feel full. Sometimes I put on my plate something that seems visually so little, but by the time I am finished it turns out that it was enough. So putting the right portion on my plate is a strategy for me so that I am not tempted to overeat. If I can do something as simple as putting less on my plate and that makes it easier, then I will do just that.

It's A Process

I think that working to become healthier is a constant learning experience and I will never get to the point where I get it just right every time. I am at the point now where I can predict if I will be over or under on the scale the next day given what I ate the day before. As I write this, I know that today I had a good day and so I will likely be pleased with the data I receive tomorrow. I have come to know what types of foods work toward me achieving my goal and what portion size is appropriate.

Digital Scale

I am glad I bought that digital scale that was on sale for $9.99

since that turned out to be a big part of my success. By weighing myself everyday at the same time I learn and see the immediate impact that eating has on my weight.

As a researcher and academic, I also find it interesting to see the impact that eating and other activities has on my weight. For example, I weigh myself at night just before going to bed and then in the morning and see how much I have lost overnight. Or before and after a bike ride. Or before and after a meal, or a glass of water, and so on.

I understand that this can be taken to the extreme and can result in obsessive compulsive disorder or as a preamble to anorexia, but this is not what I am advocating. I have done it just to better understand my body. I am tackling this as a researcher and I am simply trying to see how different actions impact my data. As I said I did each once in three months just to see what impact it had as a fun experiment, but it was not something that I plan to do again or something that I do daily or weekly or even monthly. For me it was a one time thing that I did out of curiosity because I felt that it would be interesting to know. I did it and was satisfied.

By always weighing myself in the same way, for example without clothes on, helps keep the routine consistent and gives me a more accurate read. If I weigh myself in the morning one day and then after lunch on another, obviously my numbers would vary and it would be harder for me to tell what impact my routine is having, so weighing myself every morning helps. I believe that I have set realistic goals and I understand that reaching and maintaining my goal takes time and effort. Before I started, I also knew that reaching my goal would take time. For example, between March 24th, 2015 and May 25, 2015, I lost 19 pounds. I am sure that if I wanted to I could have accelerated the process, but would I have been able to sustain it? I feel the changes I made and the way that I made them are working for me. I first cut out my weekend binge days, then I cut down on my portion size, and I changed the types of foods I eat. My diet now is not any less delicious, and I still really enjoy the foods I eat. I do not feel that I am missing out on anything and I feel better overall.

If I find that what I am doing is not working then I simply need to change what I am doing. Everyday I should be at the same weight or less than I was the day before. If I am not, then I am doing something wrong and I need to change what I am doing. My weight fluctuates by a couple of pounds but the lowest weight I am when I weigh myself should continue to be lower and lower until I reach my goal.

Goals And Milestones

I set my short-term goals from Friday to Friday. So, for example, if my lowest weight on any given Friday is 148 pounds, my goal for the following Friday could be to reach a weight that is 146 pounds or lower. Again, my scale does not lie to me, if I am not losing the weight that I expect to lose, then I am not doing it right and I need to use the data to correct my food intake and to place me back on track. If I do not reach my goal I do not beat myself up about it, but I simply become more determined.

In setting my milestones, I am much more flexible. I do not set a date but I simply set a goal and I celebrate quietly with myself when I do. So continuing with the example above, if I currently weigh 148 pounds, my next milestone would be when I reach 145 pounds. I do not specifically set a date for when I want it to happen by. I know that by focusing on my short-term goals, I will hit my milestone and when it does happen it is a very nice feeling.

When No One Is Around

I have also come to learn that, what also counts is not what I eat and do when people are around but what I eat and do when I am alone, when no one is around. I know people who can eat very little in the presence of others, but when they are alone they become human vacuum cleaners as the suck up everything in sight. Again, the scale does not lie and so if this is happening it is obvious and no one is being fooled. I often hear people say that they do not eat and yet they are overweight; I am skeptical that this is the case, especially since I have seen these very same people lose some weight in the past and then put it back on. So if they were able to lose weight in the past by eating less, then they can certainly do it now. What I mean is that if they eat less they will lose the weight. I understand that for many people food is an addiction and an illness and so being able to lose weight given that context has a different meaning. But if they did eat less, they would lose weight. Whether they can accomplish that is a different question.

What I think is that many people who try to lose weight, chose a method that is not sustainable and that resulted in not being able to make the lifestyle changes required to reach a certain goal. There are plenty of people on a diet that I know that are trying to lose weight in ways that I could never make work for me. I know myself and I know that many dieting fads and approaches I will not even attempt. Some are too complicated, others too cumbersome. In contrast, for me what I have shared throughout this book works well for me and I hope it will work well for others. Again, whatever method you chose is fine and the more options we have to chose from the more people will hopefully find an option that they can embrace.

Evidence Based

Also, some that I know are still under the illusion that exercise will compensate for their large portions; unfortunately, this has not proven to be the case, and they still keep on doing the same thing expecting a different result. The beauty of data based dieting that I am proposing is that it is evidence based and changing what I do if it is not working for me is central. I simply modify and keep changing until I get the results I desire. Ultimately, the only person that can make the changes is me. I also like that as long as I eat less, then I can eat almost anything if my goal is weight loss. My goal is better health in general and so eating less for me needs to be coupled with eating better foods.

As I keep repeating, the only way to lose weight is to eat less. How do I know how much to eat, I simply use the data that I get from the scale every morning as my tool. Remember that I can lie to others, but I cannot lie to myself. I can try and fool myself, but I cannot lie to myself, if you see the distinction I am trying to make. And once I reach my goal, I will continue to use the scale to maintain my weight.

Sometimes I have to remind myself that it's okay to feel full, as opposed to stuffed, as long as I am eating enough and the right foods. As I work to retrain my body, I now need less and less food to feel full, and I now feel that I am better (not perfect) able to trust my body to tell me when I am full and when I am hungry.

Since it is not perfect, at times I still find it hard to listen to my body when it tells me that I am full, and not to eat. At times when my body tells me that I do not need to eat I sometimes feel that I want to eat more. In these cases, walking away works. I sometimes brush my teeth, use mouthwash or do some other activity to distract me. Again, I try to always check what my body is telling me, with what my head is telling me, and if I know that I have had enough food, then I need to question what my body is telling me and to make a decision.

Again, check with a doctor or some other professional if you are unsure of how much food is enough. I cannot say this enough times, a problem is that we think way too much food is what is enough. We are so used to over eating that our bodies are trained to want more even though we do not need anymore.

The hope is that eventually, my body will be retrained and then I can return to listening to my body and use it as a guide to determine when I am hungry and how much food I need. The hope is that I will be able to trust my body again. Fortunately, we are made up of body, mind, spirit, and emotions and so we have various tools that work holistically together at our disposal. Getting them aligned is a process and not something that I can say I have achieved once and for all. As a human I am complicated and so I need to constantly work at becoming aligned.

As I said a few times, my daughters listen to their bodies; as a child I had to finish what was on my plate and so I was trained to listen to an external authority rather than my body. The result is that my body is broken and needs to be fixed. It needs to be retrained to know when to eat and how much food is enough. This is the hope I hold out for myself, that one day this will be possible and reliable.

No Wrong Way

What I have been sharing is not a recipe, but an account of what works for me. I recognize that you are not me and that if you want to try doing what I have done, then you need to use the data/scale and research what works for you. Ultimately, there is no wrong way, but the scale does not lie.

We need to continue to challenge the myths that we are trained to see as truths. When we are told not to throw out food, and to finish what is on our plate, I would argue that, in fact, it is better to throw food out than eat it, and better still to learn to buy and make less. As I shared earlier, 4 liters of milk use to last me 4 days, now it lasts weeks and I have to frequently throw out expired milk because I do not finish in weeks what used to last me days. So now I simply buy less milk or a brand with a longer expiry date.

Seeking A Community

Some might want to try this alone and some with others; some might feel intimated by showing others the number on the scale. At times I feel the need to tell people and that helps keep me honest. Some people might think I am bragging by sharing with others, but I am not; I need to tell people so that it is real for me. I am doing this and the world knows it, so there is no turning back.

Also, if you feel the need to share and do not have someone you feel comfortable sharing with, then share it with us. When I envisioned writing this book I saw it as a first step. The next is for us to connect, for us to start to transform ourselves and to help others who want to do the same. I encourage you to email me and to ask to be placed on a list so that we can come together virtually and in person. There is nothing more that I want than to help make the world a healthier place one person at a time. I can be reached at dr.carloricci@gmail.com

Exercise And Bad Diet

Again, I am exercising because I believe, as many do, that it is a part of good health, but not to lose weight. I can't have a bad diet and expect that exercise will get me out of it. All the exercise in the world will not make up for a bad diet.

Deciding On Ideal Weight

To decide what your ideal weight should be, consult with a doctor or other professional, and visit sites that calculate it for you to get an idea. I think that most people have an idea of what they want their weight goal to be.

All I can assure you of is that willed weight loss, data driven, evidence based weight loss works. I know because I am doing it.

On 8 July 2015 I reached my weight goal and the result is that I feel better. For the first time since I started this move to a healthier lifestyle I checked my blood pressure and pulse and I went from normal to optimal. Also, I have gone down 4-5 pant sizes depending on the cut and style. In the near future I have blood work and other appointment scheduled and I am hopeful that the lifestyle change I have made will be reflected in a positive way. Again, not everything will be cured by healthy eating, but it certainly cannot hurt. I believe that healthy eating will make me the healthiest me I can be, and of course that differs from person to person. I will do my part to get healthy and I will also seek the advice and assistance of professional when and as I feel I need to.

As I said throughout, I am not a dietitian or a medical doctor, but I need to become an expert in my own body and I know what makes me lose, and what makes me gain weight, and what makes me feel good. By paying attention to myself and how food impacts my weight I have become the expert I need to be in order to lose weight. One of my research interests is in how we learn best and my research and interest in how we learn best is directly transferable to all types of learning including learning about my body and how it reacts to different food types and quantities. This approach is consistent with a self-determined approach to learning and I see myself as living proof that it works for me, and I am a human, and so it will work for other humans.

Hardest Part: Dinner With Friends

As I said before, perhaps the hardest part for me to remain disciplined is when I get together with friends for dinner. Recall what happened during the three-day long weekend that I described earlier. The schedule called for me and my family to meet up with three different groups of friends on three consecutive days. This meant that there would be lots of food. After the first day (Saturday) I stood on the scale on Sunday and my weight was up. I weighed more than what I wanted to. However, knowing that was empowering and it allowed me to quickly adjust, and so on the Sunday and Monday I ate accordingly, which allowed me to quickly and painlessly get back on track.

How To Enjoy Dessert

Also, as I said earlier, it's not that I can never have dessert—that would be unsustainable, but what it does mean is that I am smart about it when I want to have some. I have to be realistic and keep my end goal in mind. One positive that came out of this is that I am now at the point where I savor food. For example, recall what I said earlier, since I wanted to try two out of three kinds of desserts, and I wanted more of one and just to try the other, I decided to have about an espresso spoon full or a small morsel, one small fork-full of one dessert, and for the other dessert to have a very thin sliver and very small portion.

Since I am having such realistic portions, I learn to savor foods and enjoy them in the moment. I find there is no need to have a large portion to be satisfied. I can taste the desserts and join in the group, and the upside is that by the end, I am not stuffed. As always, I weigh myself the next day and see if that strategy worked for me and in this case it did since my number was right on track. There is nothing like evidence to help determine whether what I am doing is working and if it is, I can feel free to use the same strategy with confidence the next time.

Making The World A Better Place

Again, one of my motivations in writing this book is to help make the world and everything in it a better place, and it is my belief that becoming healthier is a big step to help us get closer to that end. In the end, each of us has to do the work to get there, but I am hoping this book will offer a strategy that many will find useful and that it will hopefully serve to motivate many to better health. Losing weight is not easy, but it is possible and I believe that each of us can achieve healthier living. Again, if you feel good and you have no reason to lose weight, if you are healthy and happy, then keep doing what you are doing. But if you are like many of us who need to change our eating habits then there is no time like the present.

As I argue in a lot of my other writing, we can all contribute to make the world a better place. One way of doing that is to begin with ourselves. We are a part of the world and so if we become healthier, the world overall becomes a healthier place. Also, by modeling healthier living we show that it is possible and hopefully others will feel inspired to join. If there were no vegetarians, I believe it would be harder for those of us who choose to be, to do so. Living and learning from others and seeing what is possible and deciding to replicate that is contagious, and catching on to good things is positive for the individual and the world at large.

Those Whose Diets Have Failed

Almost everyone I know has tried to diet at one point or another and many have failed to sustain their diet. My point is that dieting is not easy and so rather than think of it as a diet, what works for me is to know that I am making a healthy lifestyle change. To me a diet can imply a short-term change, but a new lifestyle is permanent. Dieting and making a lifestyle change are not easy things to do. They require a strong will, but if wanted bad enough it is very possible.

In my case, I feel healthier and happier because of it. I feel better physically, mentally, emotionally, and spiritually. I also feel that I am no longer overworking my body. I feel that my body is more relaxed and that it is working at a more manageable pace. When I was throwing gluttonous amounts of extra food down my throat, my body had to work overtime to digest it all. I believe that by doing so it put a strain on my body and organs, and so much energy was put in digesting it all that less energy was available for other things. Now, I feel that my body is working at a gentler pace and I feel better for it.

Some may find it easier than others to approach and sustain moving to a healthier lifestyle, but if the will is there it can be done. Many have successfully made lifestyle changes and report feeling healthier for it. Of course, the way I did it is not the only way, and the most important thing is not what path you choose to better health, but that you achieve better health. In this case the end result is more important than the process.

For me an evidence based lifestyle change worked and it worked well, in part because I saw results immediately, which helped keep me motivated. Seeing results daily and sometimes weekly makes me want to continue. Once I reached my goal, it is still imperative that I continue to stand on the scale daily so that I can correct immediately if I get off track. This is not a onetime thing and once the goal is reached then I can go back to overeating. This is a lifelong commitment but it is sustainable. I do not find it onerous, arduous, or burdensome, but inspirational, stimulating, and rousing. This is the new me and I love it. I love that I have found a formula that works for me, that I discovered a sustainable path. I do not feel that I am missing anything. I love the food I eat and look forward to every meal because I have found a smarter way to eat that does not require me to sacrifice taste. For me now, eating is not a chore but is as delicious as ever.

Dealing With The Unexpected

Ultimately, sometimes no matter how hard I try, things do not go exactly as planned and as I would expect. When this happens I am gentle with myself and I keep moving forward. Sometimes the number on the scale does not reflect what I think should be happening, but rather than get frustrated I remain patient and keep working at what I am doing. Strangely, there have been occasions where the number remained stable for days and then suddenly dropped a few numbers overnight.

When it seems that I am not going to reach my short-term goals as I thought I would, through hard work and persistence I eventually do. I cannot always explain it and it does not always make sense but being persistent and trusting in that if I keep at it the process works, and it certainly does. Not seeing the numbers move as quickly as I would like sometimes requires persistence and patience. As I said earlier, I can usually predict what my numbers will be the next day given what I ate the day before, but sometimes it does not quite compute.

Also, when the numbers go up instead of down by a point or two, that can similarly be frustrating. When what I expect to happen does not happen I try to see that as motivation to keep at it, and since it has always eventually worked in my favor, so far, I am confident that by continuing to do what I am doing, and adjusting as the evidence demands, this approach will continue to yield positive results for me.

One thing is clear, if I give up and stop doing what I am doing, then I will never get the results I am hoping for, but if I am determined and I keep at it, I will reach my goal of achieving better health. Sometimes what I expect to happen in days, might take a week, and I have learned to accept that. My ultimate goal is what I am working toward and so as long as I move in that direction, and if my short-term goals and milestones might fluctuate a bit, then so be it.

What I know for sure is that once I hit 148 pounds, for example, it will take some time to get back to 167 pounds and I will not make that happen. However, rather than always being at 148 pounds I might hit 150 pounds and that is okay. After all having a glass of water or two can result in that type of fluctuation and so I have learned not to be discouraged by that small change. If it keeps creeping up, then I should rethink what I am doing in a more determined way, but small fluctuations and me getting back to 148 pounds is not something to worry about. In short, those types of short-term fluctuations are normal as long as in the grand scheme of things I continue to trend in the right direction.

Not Easy

I am not going to pretend that this is an easy process because it is not, and like everything else some will find it more difficult than others. Ultimately, many will abandon the goal and many will make the change. It is so difficult because in part, food is made to be addictive. The goal of capitalism is to make money and for many food manufacturers the tool to make money is food; so ultimately, I believe, that for too many manufacturers since their goal is to make money, they will stop at nothing to try and make that happen. The more we eat the more they sell; the more they sell, the more money they make; the tastier and more addictive the food, the more they will sell. In part, the drive to make more money and the addictive taste of food is what makes dieting and healthy living so difficult.

For many this will be our Everest. The best I can say is that I will be sending positive beams of energy your way, and that I believe that ultimately all of us have a strong enough will to do this. In my case, when the cravings appear too strong, that is when it is time to gather all the muster I can and to resist. I tell myself that no matter how strong the urge is to eat in an unhealthy way, if I do not eventually I will feel better for not giving in to the temptation. Eventually I realize that I am okay without it, and I am better off. The next day when I stand on the scale and I see the results, I feel even better. The best game to win is the one to better health.

Humans Can Do Incredible Things

Humans can do incredible things. If a boxer can slug it out for 12 rounds, and a climber reach Everest, and a doctor endure an 18 hour surgery, and . . . surely I can resist a chocolate bar, and I can. Very infrequently, if the craving is still too great, I feel free to have a morsel, and I am usually satisfied. All I need usually is a small taste to savor and that usually does it. Ultimately, you need to create your own strategies and whatever works for you to stave off the urges is valuable. Eating is something we should do to maintain health, not to destroy it. This book is an attempt to get us back on track to good health.

There Is An Interest

Another reason I am writing this is book is that I believe there is a need and interest in what I did. As I am losing more and more weight, and I run into people they notice that I am thinner. They ask me how I did it and I briefly share with them what I am doing. The next time I meet some of them they say that they are also trying my approach and for some it has worked and for others it has not. Some say that they are standing on the scale everyday. I remind them that merely standing on a scale everyday is not going to result in becoming healthier. The scale is a tool and the secret is eating smarter by having smaller portions, if your portions are currently too large, and eating healthier foods if what you are currently eating is not. Again, at times becoming healthier is hard and requires a strong will, but it is not impossible. In fact, it is very possible and the reward is a healthier mind, body, spirit, and emotions—well worth the effort.

People sometimes ask me "what if I do this?" or "what if I do that?" will I get to my goal of a healthy weight? For example, they might ask, "If I eat the same portion sizes, but of healthier food, would I get to my healthy weight?" My response is usually, I do not really know if it will work, I then encourage them to try it, and then to stand on the scale and to use that actual information to answer their question based on evidence, and to use that data to guide them.

Is Being Unhealthy A Sickness?

For many of us leading an unhealthy lifestyle and eating unhealthy foods and portions is a sickness, fortunately one that we can treat, sometimes not easily, but we can treat it. This book is a story about what I have done to treat myself and how I put myself on a road to better health. I know that because I feel healthier, and other evidence is suggesting that I am healthier.

The idea is to lose weight, but also to eat smarter, and healthier, and if I am often binging and still losing weight, I do not see that as me eating smarter and healthier. Having said that, I am only human and if I have lapses then I should forgive myself, and simply get back on track right away, and continue to try and do things that will reduce the frequency and excess of my lapses. Lapsing feels awful but getting back on track and seeing the number I want to see on the scale feels awesome.

The theory behind becoming healthier that I have outlined is very simple, the execution, admittedly and I know from living it, can be much more challenging, but possible. I hear reasons for why people cannot lose weight, and some say it's because of their metabolism, or their thyroid, or that they are not eating all that much and so on. I am not saying this to be critical or to disparage those who try and fail to get healthier, but I sincerely mean it to be supportive, we all can lose weight. Granted, the reasons above and many others might make things more difficult, but becoming healthier is still possible. There are not very many things that apply universally to all of the billions of people on the earth, but this, I believe, does: If you eat less then you will lose weight. Also, granted, what constitutes "less" varies from person to person, but the rule still applies.

There is a certain threshold that applies to each of us and it might vary from day to day, or year to year, or decade to decade, but if we eat more we will gain weight, if we eat at that threshold we will remain the same weight, and if we eat less we will lose weight. How do you know where you stand on the threshold? The answer is simple: Stand on the scale and it will reveal all.

The scale does not discriminate. It treats everyone the same. No matter who stands on the scale it will not lie. I am learning to eat to be healthy, and not to excess, or ill-health.

After reading a draft of the book here is what a nurse who specializes in nutrition wrote back to me:

"Being a primary healthcare provider for 500 patients, I am solely responsible for their health management, which includes health teaching related to diet and exercise. I appreciate your stance on this process of weight loss being a lifestyle change rather than a diet. For most people, small milestones are key and those changes have to be addressed as a life style modification rather than a diet because they are just that—an adjustment and improvement to their old unhealthy ways. The word diet implies short term rather than a means to a healthier way of life and therefore it holds more significance when outlined as a modification or life change. To make healthy choices is key in weight management. Having said that I also feel that food intake has to be realistic, smaller portions yes, but the caloric intake also has to be enough to sustain your daily activities. In terms of a health standpoint, your book raises very good points that weight management is associated with healthy food portions."

Growing A Community

I hope you find what I have done worthwhile, inspirational, and easy enough to replicate. I hope I have made the simplicity of it clear, and that you feel you can become healthier by following a similar path, or any other that you feel might work better for you. If you need clarification on something or motivation then please send me an email and I will try and help as best I can. Also, I will send you notices of events and gatherings that may happen online or face-to-face. I think if we are going to do this, then we need to create a community of committed and supportive people. We need to stay in touch and share our stories so that we can continue to help ourselves and to help others who might be looking for something similar. If you like, I can be reached at dr.carloricci@gmail.com. Again, hope to hear from you soon and best of luck in your journey to better health.

In Five Easy Steps

Finally, here is a summary in five easy steps of what I have outlined throughout the book:

1. Decide that you want and need to lose weight to get

healthy.

2.   Decide how much weight you need to lose to get healthy.

3.   Begin to eat smarter by, for example, eating smaller portions and healthier foods.

4.   Stand on the scale every day to determine if what you are doing is helping you to reach your long-term goal to better health.

5.   Repeat steps one to five on your way to better health.

7 EPILOGUE

From July 15th to August 12th we were away from home. During that time I did not have access to my scale; nevertheless, I stuck to my new eating approach and hoped for continued success. When I left for my trip I had already reached my weight goal I set for myself and was working toward. Admittedly, since I was feeling great at that weight, I was a little worried about not having a scale while away. While on vacation, I did think about what a scale would reveal when I finally would get a chance to step on one. While away I did think of asking the hotels if they had one, and I even thought about going into a box-store and taking one off the shelf to weigh and see, but I did not. In fact, I even passed a public scale a few times by chance, once at a restaurant entrance and another time at a mall, but for some reason I still did not weigh myself.

In planning for my time away I did pack some healthy snacks and favorite non-perishable foods such a nuts, chickpeas, dried fruit, and my breakfast cereal, and I am glad that I did. It helped me stay on track because it was not always convenient to get healthy food. Having said that, usually with not too much effort, I was able to get healthy options almost at will. Fresh fruit, oatmeal, yogurts, veggie sandwiches, tacos, and other healthy options were available. But having the food with me readily available made it much, much more convenient.

We also ate in our room and rented places with kitchenettes whenever possible, which it was for more than half of our trip. We prefer eating at home and cooking our own meals. My daughters protest when we have to eat out and cheer when we are able to return to home cooking.

In short, when I returned home from our trip, the next morning I continued my routine and so I stepped on my scale for the first time in over a month, very curious to see what it would reveal. I felt that I was on track and in fact the scale confirmed that.

Since then, I continue to weigh myself and I am finding that I am in a great rhythm. I am getting better and better at doing the things that I need to do to remain healthy and at my goal weight. I still have very reasonable portion sizes and stand on the scale to weigh and see whether I am where I want to be.

I still want to balance healthy eating with weight control. Remember that a big part of my objective is to eat healthier more nutritious foods and keep my weight in check, I am still very conscious of eating healthier options and not overindulging on unhealthy foods is a big part of that for me.

I recently attending a family barbeque and there were two dessert options and I tried them both. I took the original piece they gave me and I went back to the host and told her that it was too big for me and asked if she minded if I cut my own piece. Of course she did not mind and I put what I thought was reasonable on my plate and I ate it and was satisfied. Then unbeknownst to me they brought out a second dessert which is among my favorite and so I had a little of that as well.

The next day when I stood on the scale I was up only modestly since I mostly kept my portion sizes in check. So since I was up, that day, I adjusted accordingly and by the following day I was back on track.

I also find that I am getting better at listening to my body and that I stop eating when I am full. Recently my daughters wanted pizza and so we ordered it. They prefer just cheese and I wanted sundried tomatoes on mine, so I ordered a one topping pizza with the topping on the side. I was planning to have one slice but halfway through I realized that between the pizza and all of the sundried tomatoes I was full half-way through eating my very large slice. I stopped, placed the leftovers in a Tupperware and simply had it the next day. In the past I would have ploughed through even though I was full and likely even had another slice, and another.

I understand that this is a lifelong process and that I will continue to refine and add better and more nutritious foods to my diet, and sometimes not so nutritious ones. For example, I now add flaxseed and Blackstrap Molasses to my shake and I have a greater variety of nuts, usually as a morning snack.

I have always liked fruit but I have come to really, really love it. It is so sweet and delicious and sometimes while I am eating it, I find it hard to believe how nutritious and good it is for me. I am used to thinking that if it tastes so good, it's because it is bad for you, but that is not always the case, nutritious food can also be tasty food.

Another strategy that I have come to rely on is that when I go out I bring healthy food options with me if I know I am going to be away for an extended period. For example, I am taking my dad to a doctor's appointment today and so I have fresh and dried fruit, and a veggie sandwich. This way when I feel the need I can eat and I am not scrambling to find food, and I am not scrambling to find healthy options. If I have food with me, I find that it also makes life less stressful. When I am hungry food is there, and I do not have to rush around and detour to get some.

I have come to realize that no diet will allow me to eat more, and that no diet will allow me to eat unhealthy foods, if my goal is to maintain my weight and get healthier. The bottom line is that getting healthier requires that I eat more nutritious foods and that I eat less. Many people that I speak to seem to be looking for a magic wand that will allow them to eat a lot and even non-nutritious foods. They seem to hope that if they cut out this or that, and eat only certain foods that then they will lose weight, for example. Or if they walk so many steps or exercise for so long and burn so many calories, that then they could indulge and still lose weight and get healthier. Unfortunately, this is not the case. No matter how much some of us would wish it, no healthy diet will recommend or include eating a bag of chips every night.

Also, when I first started, if I was only losing 1 or 2 pounds by the end of the month I believe I would have needed to reassess. Also, when I look at my current weight and consider my short term and long-term goals, if overall I gained 10 pounds by the end of the month but lost 2 pounds along the way, I have to be honest with myself and say that I am up 8 pounds not down 2. That is where keeping long term and short term goals in mind comes into play.

In addition, if I stand on the scale only once a week I might be tempted to eat like mad for a few days and then to starve myself to make a certain weight, once again I would have to be honest with myself and admit that something is not working.

For me getting healthier requires and necessitates eating nutritious foods almost exclusively, and eating the correct amount of food per day. Short of this there is no pill or magic wand that will work, but the great thing, I have discovered, is that there is something I can do that does work, and that has become painless and, in fact, beneficial for me.

I have come to realize that, simply put, overeating will result in weight gain, and eating less nutritious foods will diminish and not optimize my health.

To date, I have told very few people about my method to better health and a few of those I have told have shared with me that they tried the weigh and see approach. Of those a few have said that it is not for them, nor have they adopted another approach and they have continued with the status quo. I assume that they are not ready or willing to lose weight or that they are happy with where they currently are and that is fine.

Working your way to better health is not something that is easy and some will find it more challenging than others, but once embraced and the results start to manifest, many will be thrilled with the results. I know I am and so are many that I have talked to who have become healthier using whatever approach worked for them. As well, those who do not sustain the results, seem disappointed as a result.

Of the few I have shared the approach with, some have reported success. Recently one person shared with me that she felt that she overate and felt that the scale would confirm it when she stood on it, and indeed that was the case. From one day to the next the scale read 4 pounds higher than the day before. The fact that she stood on the scale daily helped her confirm that and to quickly get back on track. The immediate data and evidence worked to confirm and correct her lapse quickly. She shared that the weigh and see approach is helping. I can only hope that many, many others will also find better health by adopting it.

I have no doubt that everyone will get results if they stick to the approach outlined in this book. Again, I know that it is not easy, but it is possible. In my case I realize that it is ultimately up to me to stick to it and I am glad that I am and can only work to ensure that I will continue. I am finding it easier and easier to do so and I hope that will continue to be the case. Eating this way is the way I now eat and I keep reminding myself of that.

To end the book, I have left 7 pages (one for each day of the week) where you can document what you eat in the morning, afternoon, and evening. You can then share this information with a professional or simply use it as a reminder of what you ate that day. Following that, I have left a few pages where you can jot down notes. Feel free to use it to note questions, comments, reminders and so on.

Date:

Morning:

Afternoon:

Evening:

Date:

Morning:

Afternoon:

Evening:

Date:

Morning:

Afternoon:

Evening:

Date:

Morning:

Afternoon:

Evening:

Date:

Morning:

Afternoon:

Evening:

Date:

Morning:

Afternoon:

Evening:

Date:

Morning:

Afternoon:

Evening:

Notes:

Notes:

ABOUT THE AUTHOR

Carlo Ricci, PhD is a full Professor at the Schulich School of Education, Nipissing University, Graduate Studies. He founded and edits the *Journal of Unschooling and Alternative Learning* (*JUAL*). He has published a number of books and articles. Among the books he has written and edited are, *Turning Points: 35 Educational Visionaries in Education Tell Their Own Stories* (co-edited with Jerry Mintz) (2010); *The Willed Curriculum, Unschooling, and Self-Direction: What Do Love, Trust, Respect, Care, and Compassion Have To Do With Learning?* (2012); *The Legacy of John Holt: A Man Who Genuinely Understood, Trusted, and Respected* Children (co-edited with Pat Farenga) (2013); *Natural Born Learners: Unschooling and Autonomy in Education* (co-edited with Beatrice Ekwa Ekoko (2014)); *Holistic Pedagogy: The Self and Quality Willed Learning* (Springer Press 2015) (co-authored with Conrad Pritscher).

His research interests include Unschooling; Homeschooling; Holistic Education; Self-determined Learning; Free Schools; Democratic Schools; Online Learning; Technology and Learning; Play; Natural Learning; Curiosity; Healthy Lifestyle; Willed Learning; and the Willed Curriculum.